# Guide for Caregivers

**Keeping Your Spirit Healthy When Your Caregiver Duties and Responsibilities Are Dragging You Down**

# Benjamin Pratt

*Nancy and Ed,*
*With a deep sense of*
*admiration, gratitude and*
*affection,*
*Benjamin,*
*October, 2011*

---

## Read The Spirit Books

an imprint of
David Crumm Media, LLC
Canton, Michigan

For more information and further discussion, visit
**http://www.GuideForCaregivers.com**

Cover art and design by
Rick Nease
www.RickNeaseArt.com



Published By
Read The Spirit Books
an imprint of
David Crumm Media, LLC
42015 Ford Rd., Suite 234
Canton, Michigan, USA



For information about customized editions, bulk pur-
chases or permissions, contact David Crumm Media, LLC at
info@DavidCrummMedia.com

# Contents

## PART 6

# Dedication

DEDICATED TO JUDITH—MY WIFE, companion and friend of 48 years who is a gifted caregiver and a resilient, feisty care receiver.

# Preface

HOW DO YOU CARE for yourself when you feel you are taking care of the rest of the world? If you are experiencing the joys and sorrows and the ups and downs of caregiving, this book is for you. It is for parents for whom parenting may never end because a child is physically, emotionally or intellectually disabled; it is for parents with a child who has returned home because of a physical, mental or intellectual condition that prevents independent living; it is for spouses caring for loved ones because of some disabling condition; it is for adults who are caring for parents, often as part of the sandwich generation.

This book is intended to restore a new and right spirit in you. Our goal is to restore balance to your spirit—to replace sadness with laughter, fear with hope, exhaustion with vitality, mourning with gratitude, emptiness with joy and burnout with a rekindled passion.

Every caregiver is unique. Every care receiver is unique. Every caregiver/care receiver relationship is unique as are the stresses and successes, joys and sorrows, anxious and serene moments in each relationship. What is not unique is the basic necessity of each caregiver to maintain *self*—body and soul.

Only by accomplishing this can you continue to care in optimal fashion for your loved one.

This book will help you to identify with women and men who give of body, mind and soul to care for the well-being of one or more persons. There are professional caregivers—doctors, nurses, clergy, physical therapists, etc.; and there are informal caregivers—usually family and friends who give brief or around-the-clock care of loved ones with:

- Emotional or mental problems
- Dilemmas associated with aging
- Developmental disabilities (physical, emotional or intellectual)
- Physical illness and related limitations

This book offers guidance for the basic necessities of sustaining both your body and your soul. It is full of life-living wisdom garnered from folks who have walked the walk, lived the life, suffered the defeats, felt the agonies and the boredom, extended the compassion with a gentle word or a tender touch, experienced anger and frustration, celebrated the joys and depths of meaning and purpose, relaxed with the laughter, felt mortality and immortality—the limitations of our mortal bodies and the boundless yearnings of our unquenchable spirits.

This book will give you permission to feel, to think and to express the wide range of emotions, yearnings, fears and desires that are yours as a caregiver.

# PART 1

## Getting Started

# CHAPTER 1

# Measuring Our Spirit

## My Voice...

This is a book for your spirit. Is your spirit joyous? Are you filled with hope? Do you have energy—mental, physical, and sexual? Do you play and laugh? Are you just enduring? Are you dull? Does "exhausted" describe you? Do you sometimes feel brittle and broken? Are you bitter and cynical? Were you once 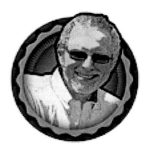 on fire and now burned out? As a caregiver, these are important and not easily answered questions. You could probably name many other descriptions of your spirit. **Jot them down, please** ! Yes, you will want a pencil or pen while reading this book.

I hope to help you individually or jointly to craft practices of the heart, mind and body that will enable you to yearn for and move toward the day when you can say with gratitude that your life is good as it is given. The Psalmist poetically crafted our yearning:

"Create in me a clean heart, O God, and put a new and right spirit within me."

—*Psalm 51:10*

How do we get there? How do we prevent or restore a broken, burned out, exhausted and cynical spirit? The problem is a spiritual one. Please remember that. I'm not providing medical or psychological solutions. This book is about finding spiritual solutions to cope with your life as a caregiver.

To sustain or restore your spirit you will be making a spiritual journey. But let me be very clear about that phrase. Spirituality seeks to answer three questions, not so much by reason and intellect, as by forging the answers from the bricks we craft and bake through our daily living. These questions of spirituality are:

- Why should I climb out of bed in the morning?
- How can I make it through another tiring, exhausting, stressful day?
- And, at the end of the day, did I do anything that really matters; not for all of humankind, but in my small, task-driven world?

You answer these daily by living the extraordinary life you live as a caregiver of your loved one. It is right there in the care of your loved one that you answer through your hands, heart, lips, mind, eyes and soul. It is there that your spirit is restored and sustained—or broken and burned out. These are nuts and bolts questions that ground us. As they often say in AA: "Religion is for people who try to stay out of hell. Spirituality is for those of us who have already been there."

A professor who helped to pack my spiritual parachute often said, "There are two primary ingredients necessary to be a religious or spiritual person—honesty and imagination." In these chapters, I am giving you a wide range of the open and honest yearnings, hopes, fears, angers, frustrations, joys and imaginative statements by persons who have lived the life of a caregiver. I have recorded some comments as free verse. I have also given you plenty of white space to jot, scribble, and struggle with yourself as you experience these utterances. Given the rigor of your schedule, you won't have time to do this all at once! Take it at your own pace. Remember, you can't push a string, or your own soul!

A word of **caution** ! Don't do this alone. By that I mean: If you take this seriously, and I hope you will, this process is likely to stir deep feelings in you, so you will need a very good friend who will sit down with you and listen to your story and feelings and confusion. Or you may want to speak with a pastor or a counselor. This is all about restoring your spirit so that you can care for your beloved.

What are the bricks we must craft and bake through our daily living to restore our burned out, cynical heart—to craft a clean heart? We need to tell our story with honesty, integrity and respect to someone whom we deeply trust.

## Wisdom of the Community...

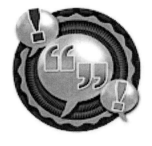

"You know that BP Oil CEO, Tony 'Somebody,' who whined that he wanted to get his life back? A lot of people got real pissed at ol' Tony. I thought a lot about that statement of his—I got angry at him but I also felt some sympathy for him.

"Since my son got wounded, I have often thought how I wish we could get our life back—you know, as it was—comfortable, simple, and familiar. I often felt angry or jealous as well as guilty for thinking I wanted my life back. I guess the difference between ol' Tony and us is that he is paid the big bucks to prevent the unexpected. The unexpected just happened to us and we are coping. We are on the front line—in the trenches, all day, every day. This is our life!

"A lot of folks on the Gulf Coast wish they could get their lives back also. The unexpected in their lives was caused by the failures of various people, Tony being one of them. Regardless, whether we caused it or someone else caused it, our lives have to be lived as best we can. Our son was doing his job when that damn bomb went off. None of us will ever get back to the life we had. One thing feels pretty strange to me now—I've never felt more like I have a reason to stay alive than I do now."

—*The parent of a disabled veteran*

"How do I begin to restore myself and let some refreshing waters flow into my soul? How can I begin to revitalize myself so that I might feel some joy and fewer burdens as I live the life of a sacrificial giver?"

—*A longtime caregiver*

"Attitude is a little thing that makes a big difference."

—*Sir Winston Churchill*

"Courage is more exhilarating than fear and in the long run it is easier. We do not have to be heroes overnight."

"Do one thing every day that scares you."

—*Eleanor Roosevelt*

"Many people will walk in and out of your life, but only true friends will leave footprints in your heart."

—*Unknown author*

"I have noticed even people who claim everything is predestined and that we can do nothing to change it look before crossing the road."

—*Scientist Stephen Hawking from the perspective of life in a wheelchair, physically dependent on a caregiver*

"Do I feel out of control? Yes! Am I different than I used to be? Yes! Do I resent this task? Yes! Some of the time I get very resentful or openly angry! Do I feel ashamed of these feelings? Yes! And that really perplexes me. It doesn't make any sense. It is as if I feel responsible and guilty that this is the direction our life has gone!"

—*A caregiver*

---

"I'm **only** a husband! I suspect most caregivers are initially treated like a god, with superpower. Then we become invisible. I'm not a superman. I'm a responsible, very fragile, determined caregiver with a wide range of feelings from tender compassion to anger."

—*A caregiver*

---

"I learned how to educate others about how best to work with me. I have found that I have had to teach many people I meet how to provide accommodations, how to help me learn, how to see past my wheelchair! This gets me back to my main point: If we could take the 'special' out of education and just focus on giving all kids an education, I don't think it would be so complicated for students with disabilities to grow up and be successful adults. Bottom line: We aren't that special—we want a life like yours!"

—*A young woman with cerebral palsy (CP)*

---

"I suspect many caregivers feel like I do—that I had to go on stage without ever having a dress rehearsal. This is improv theatre and I'm winging it. Where is my script? Where is my rehearsal?"

—*A caregiver*

---

# Let's Get Your Spirit Ready for a New Day

**Some questions to ponder and answer...**

Do you yearn for your previous life?

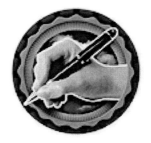

Do you feel jealous of others?

Do you feel a sense of purpose? When does that arise in you? What reminds you of your purpose?

**Read the following words and jot down ways you experience each one:**

Angry

Broken

Burned out

Guilty

Sad

Cynical

# CHAPTER 2

# Using This Book

I suspect that if you have just finished "Measuring Your Spirit," you are puzzled and curious to now find a chapter on how to use this book. Why now, Benjamin? This seems out of order—should it not have come first? Well, you would think so, except in the life of a caregiver. Caregivers often experience life out of order. Life gives us the test before we even sign up for the course, certainly before we have a chance to study and learn what to do as a caregiver. The least I can do is explain what to expect as you turn the pages of this book.

In truth, though, this is the correct order. You began by taking an assessment of your spirit. The remainder of this book is filled with practices to guide, restore, sustain and protect your spirit as a caregiver.

WE HAVE TAKEN THE loud and clear advice of caregivers and care receivers: **Make these readings short!** Given the daily pace and stress of these long-term relationships, few people have time to sit down and read at length. So, as we move together toward a healthier, stronger and ultimately more joyous spiritual life, we have designed this book as a series of short passages you can pick up and read—almost anywhere the book's pages fall open. One segment at a time may be all you can manage. That is fine. After all, this is now your book.

The book is arranged in parts to make it easy to find the overall subject that most interests you. Within these parts are several chapters that zero in on specific ideas to jump-start your spiritual life. Within each chapter, you'll find three or four distinct sections.

First, each chapter opens with "My Voice." Here, I introduce the basic idea you'll find in the following few pages. I'm drawing on my experience both as a veteran counselor, a researcher who has listened to a lot of men and women in caregiving relationships while preparing this book and as a veteran caregiver myself. This first section is written both to encourage and to quickly introduce you to each new idea.

Second, each chapter includes the section called "Wisdom of the Community," which is packed with short passages from folks like you who have lived in caregiving relationships. There are occasional bits of pithy wisdom from sages, some of them famous. Mostly, though, you'll find honest, unvarnished voices of people giving and receiving care—to reassure you that you're not alone, no matter what you're experiencing right now. You'll notice that individual names have been removed from many of these real-life statements from ordinary men and women. Instead, I've marked these passages with a phrase to describe the person, such as: "a long-term caregiver." This protects the privacy of those sharing these sometimes deeply personal insights. Some of these statements are my own, written as a long-term caregiver myself. Some of them were contributed by individuals. Some of these statements from men and women were revised to combine very similar thoughts from more than one contributor. All have the sharp-edged honesty of experience.

Finally, each chapter closes with one or both of the sections called "Let's Get Your Spirit Ready for a New Day" and "Let's Imagine". The first of these is a place for your voice to emerge. Here, we've added a little white space to the book's pages in the print edition so you can actually jot down some of your own feelings, yearnings, joys, disappointments and also ideas you want to share. Yes, that's right! Keep a pen or pencil handy. I'm encouraging you to write in these pages. If you are reading this as an e-book, you might use a separate notebook, or use the note-taking feature of your book reader. If you've got an idea or insight that you think may help others, we urge you to visit our website for this book and share your ideas with other readers. In sparking your responses in this section of each chapter, I take two distinct approaches. First, in most chapters, I simply ask you questions. Please, take a moment and respond. Then, in some chapters, there is a fourth section where I sketch a scene that will be familiar to many caregivers—a scene of two friends who meet regularly for coffee and talk over the most urgent issues in their lives. This section is called "Let's Imagine," and I hope you'll enjoy it as one more avenue to get your own creative voice flowing.

Even though I am a United Methodist pastor and I write from the perspective of a pastoral counselor, this book is intended for persons of all faiths. I am here human-to-human, without bias for religious preference. My hope is that your religious or spiritual tradition will be relevant and helpful in your personal journey as a caregiver.

Hopefully, this will be a companion book, not to be read at one time or even sequentially, but as you have time and need and desire. It can be used as a guide for group study or individual exploration. I offer a few suggestions about forming a study group in the book's final chapter, "Forming a Study Group." At the end of the book, you'll also find "Resources" and some useful definitions of "burnout" and "accidie." Please take the time to read the definitions of these two often misunderstood words.

My hope is that this book will stir your heart, confront your mind, and comfort your soul. Above all, I pray that it will sustain and restore your spirit as you seek to love your beloved.

# PART 2
## Telling Our Story

# CHAPTER 3

# Talking Honestly; Listening Intently

## My Voice...

My mother died at age 63 from complications related to hip surgery that resulted in a fatal stroke. My father, an excellent auto mechanic with very little formal education, modeled how to get through his significant loss. He told his story, never intrusively, but with heartfelt sadness and a bit of fear to those 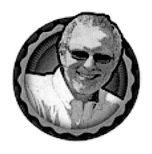 who would listen—to friends and even to some strangers. He told his story over and over until he was able to smile, even laugh again. He was a quiet, gentle country man who innately walked toward healing his deep personal loss by telling and retelling his story.

In the spring of 2010, a woman very dear to us was diagnosed with pancreatic cancer. She died 16 days after being diagnosed. Her family and friends, especially her husband, were all in shock and deep grief. Shortly after the funeral, he and I began meeting regularly at a bagel shop for coffee, bagels and conversation. What we did some of the time was talk about baseball or politics. What we did most of the time was share our respective stories about our journeys with our spouses. The telling of our stories led each of us to the recovery of long-forgotten memories—the sweet and the not so sweet. We were open and honest and respectful and confidential. We were a gift to each other through telling and listening to our stories.

The "Let's Imagine" sections of this book reflect my joys and struggles as a caregiver along with input from many others in caregiving relationships. I have formatted "Let's Imagine" to capture the spirit of those bagel and coffee mornings with my good friend. Feel free to change the menu or the setting as you envision such scenes, but use those sections to get your own voice flowing. You may want to try to establish such a real life friendship yourself.

Caregivers need a community—whether two or ten people—in which we can tell our story; a community where we are heard, validated and respected for the journey we are taking. A group of people is not necessarily a true community. Community forms when we have shared and listened to each other's stories and become aware that in spite of our differences, there is a common story that unites us. An important part of forming a caring community is not leaving anyone behind.

Good listeners are hard to find. The number one attribute and gift of a good listener is not the ear—it is the heart. A good listener has a loving, hospitable heart. Hospitality is being filled with enough love to welcome a friend or stranger into your space, to be more interested in the friend or stranger than in yourself and your agenda. Hospitality makes space to truly listen to the other's story. The listener's agenda is not primary; the storyteller's agenda is.

Hospitality demands only discerning comments as one listens. The listener basically invites clarification and does not offer judgment or advice. If I am a hospitable listener I want to know the whole story—I want to assist only by quietly inviting the story into it fullest form. The artistry of listening is this: We hear the words beneath the spoken words. We hear a voice speaking from our companion's eyes, even if our friend cannot yet voice that emerging feeling. The ability to tenderly invite the teller to focus on the unspoken is an art developed over a long journey of offering hospitality.

"If one gives answer before he hears, it is his folly and shame."
—*Proverbs 18:13.*

Good listeners are hard to find. But good listening is essential to help each other through the challenges of endless caregiving. It is a vital skill for the formation of community.

## Wisdom of the Community...

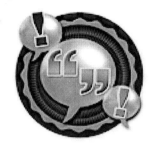

"You keep asking me how I am coping with this caregiver task. I had a thought about it the other day. Sometimes I think I think too much. Anyway, I cleaned the skin and fat off chicken on Saturday to prepare supper. I put the scraps in a couple of plastic bags and then in the trash. It's been real hot and the trash men don't come until Tuesday. By Monday, it was foul opening the trash can—it reeked. I guess that's a good metaphor of my life: Life can begin to stink very quickly. A spouse suddenly has cancer or Alzheimer's; a child is suddenly disabled or mentally ill and moves back home; a daughter gets cancer; a stroke leaves your spouse of 46 years marginally functional. These are all real for me and people in my life—it stinks!! I'm coping and trying to learn this new job of caregiver. …I'm trying hard."

—*A caregiver*

---

"Our child has made great progress in his recovery. I know he will always have problems because of the brain damage, but I think he can get a job and make his own way. More than anything else I wish he could find someone who loves him as much as we do, who would even marry him and care for him in the future."

—*A parent*

---

"I want to tell someone how difficult life is with my son. I have this grown son who has returned to our home because he is mentally ill and I am having a hell of a time coping with him. I tried to talk about my struggle with my men's group at church. I must not do it well because, within a few minutes, they are telling me about things from their lives and it never gets back to me. So, I just get quiet and listen or drift away."

—*A father*

---

"Two Travellers were on the road together, when a Bear suddenly appeared on the scene. Before he observed them, one made for the side of the road, and climbed up into the branches and hid. The other was not so nimble as his companion; and, as he could not escape, he threw himself on the ground and pretended to be dead. The Bear came up and sniffed all round him, but he kept perfectly still and held his breath: for they say that a bear will not touch a dead body. The Bear took him for a corpse, and went away. When the coast was clear, the Traveller in the tree came down, and asked the other what it was the Bear had whispered to him when he put his mouth to his ear. The other replied, "He told me never again to travel with a friend who deserts you at the first sign of danger."

—*Aesop's Fables*

---

"I'm going out to clean the pasture spring;
I'll only stop to rake the leaves away
(And wait to watch the water clear, I may):
I sha'n't be gone long.—You come too.
I'm going out to fetch the little calf
That's standing by the mother. It's so young,
It totters when she licks it with her tongue.
I sha'n't be gone long.—You come too."

—*Robert Frost*

## Let's Get Your Spirit Ready for a New Day

Name two people who share their stories with you.

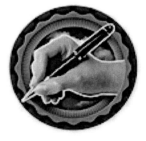

With whom do you share your story?

What have you learned about talking—and listening?

What do you do when you tell your story and get another story back rather than a hospitable response to yours?

What tips can you share about telling your story or listening to another person's story? Other readers would appreciate reading your tips, if you'd care to share them at our website [www.GuideForCaregivers.info].

# Let's Imagine

You and I have seen each other a few times but have never been introduced. It was by coincidence that we encountered each other on the street. You were hurrying along with an old friend of mine, but the two of you stopped and she introduced us. It was she who casually slipped this into the introduction: 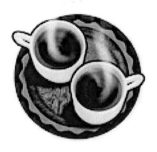 "You two people have something in common—you are both caregivers."

So, now a few weeks later, we are sitting in the shade of a pin oak tree outside a small café. A pleasant breeze adds protection from the heat. We seem to be at ease with each other—even feel trust that enables me to say: "My wife has been sick for the last seven years—severe, disabling migraines—sometimes for days on end. Recently she has had a cancer scare, followed by three surgeries. It has been very difficult for both of us. It took me a long time to clearly see how deeply it was affecting me."

After you respond with sympathetic words, you trust me with your personal story as a caregiver. Jot down an outline of the story you would tell:

# CHAPTER 4

# Risking Love

## My Voice...

Caregivers live a dangerous life of love. Love is always risky, but this deep form of love lived out by caregivers is dangerous—always prone to injury in so many forms. If you don't want to be hurt, then don't risk giving your heart to any living creature—human or animal. Be a Scrooge who lives only to make 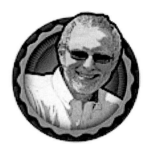 money or immerse yourself in hobbies or luxuries. Live only for yourself. If you love, your heart *will* be broken— **period** !!

As caregivers, you take love to a deeper level, risking a total commitment of your life. You are amazingly faithful, courageous—and often sacrificial, vulnerable, lonely, stressed and overburdened.

Life has asked you a very difficult question, which you have answered with your love and your life—for your loved one, your beloved. As Zora Neale Hurston said, "There are years that ask questions and years that answer."

You chose to live this vulnerability of love every day, every month—for years on end. Your loved one's physical, emotional, mental or intellectual limitations dictate the reality of the tasks you assume. Your responsibility now shapes every moment of your waking hours—and your often restless sleep as well. Time breaks down into seconds, minutes—and more often than not— relief that each hour has passed, that challenges were met and all is good for a few moments.

We can't often control the dictates of the situation, but we can muster the strength and courage to care for ourselves so we can continue to care for our loved one. Our focus here in this book is the care of ourselves as caregivers. Anyone living this life—whether the informal caregiver or the professional—will face the majority of these issues: how much to do alone; the value of community support; the value of support groups and advocacy groups; the need to examine our personal story and its implications for our ability to respond as a caregiver; and of course, burnout. It's all part of the emotional, intellectual, physical and spiritual life of a caregiver.

Here is a portion of a conversation I had with a full-time caregiver struggling with these unexpected demands in her life:

**Benjamin Pratt** : *Thank you for inviting me to visit with you. I am pleased that our mutual acquaintance arranged this conversation. She told me that you are the primary caregiver for your son who had a horrible accident and has been in a coma for many months. Did she tell you about me and what I am doing?*

**A caregiver** : *She did tell me about you and your work. I'm not sure I'm a person you want to talk to since you are a priest. I used to attend Mass all the time, but I don't anymore. Especially, since this happened.*

**Benjamin** : *From what your friend said about your tireless dedication to your son, I think you are definitely who I want to talk with. Please say more about your idea that I might not want to talk to you.*

**caregiver** : *I used to believe in God and attend Mass all the time. Since my son was in this horrific accident, I don't want anything to do with a God who would let this happen, a God who still hasn't done anything to make him better.*

**Benjamin** : *That makes perfect sense to me. You and I must have been taught the same belief—that God is all-powerful! You and a lot of other caregivers have been bewildered by this belief in the face of the condition of their loved one.*

**caregiver** : *So, if it makes sense to you, why do you stay in the church?*

**Benjamin** : *That's a question many people have asked through the centuries. I don't have an easy answer, but I think it comes down to whether we were taught that God mainly is this all-powerful force. There is another way to think about God—as all-loving. And, that's how I see God now—God is a lover, who loves us even through the limitations of what God can do in our world. There's a big difference in those two perspectives. Tell me more about what you do for your son.*

**caregiver** : *I pretty much live with him round the clock. I sleep next to him, I bathe, clean, exercise his muscles, change his diapers. I talk to him, sing to him, caress him, keep loving him in those tender ways and hoping that someday my son that I played with and enjoyed will return to his old self. I do all I can do and then I hope and sometimes cry and then hope again. I don't give up caring for him.*

**Benjamin** : *You may not think in this language, but you are, for your son, the very loving god who experiences the limitations of your power. Like God, you are a lover who gives your all. People like you keep me believing in a God whose son died loving us. Neither was all-powerful but both are lovers. That's what keeps me going. Sounds like that is what keeps you going.*

**caregiver** (after a long pause): *Yes, I am a lover of my son .*

## Wisdom of the Community...

"I'm planning to keep my wife in our home as long as I can—as long as I have the money and the stamina I'm going to keep her at home. For better or worse, you know!"

—*A husband*

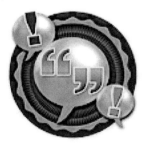

"I have become consumed by my _____'s condition. I can't seem to think of anything else—I don't seem to ever relax. I seldom read and I used to enjoy that a lot. I seldom get into my garden—most of the time I isolate myself. I guess I'm pretty damned depressed. I've lost myself and I don't know how to find me."

*—A caregiver*

---

"Yes, I'm a home care worker—that's my job or I should say one of my jobs. I enjoy caring for people. I come to love them and they need me and love me and that feels very good. But I don't have health insurance. The work is physically hard and I wonder how long I can do it before I wear out. I don't make much money. I haven't had a raise in I don't know when."

*—A professional caregiver*

---

"My husband was dying. My whole world was focused on him, not on myself. What right did I have to feel sorry for myself? In fact, I never thought or felt it until I crawled exhausted into bed, my lonely bed. All that attention on him kept me from facing a lot of things I must have been holding too close to the bone to let them be felt."

*—A wife*

---

"I have been hurt too many times. I want a predictable, comfortable place where I feel in control. Oh, I know the cost of safety may be boredom and a life of regrets. It is safer to be an 'unhappy hoper' and an 'unhappy rememberer' than to risk the cost of embracing the elusive promise of love. I can't trust others enough to risk embracing the promise of joy."

*—A caregiver*

"I don't know what to say when he talks about such difficult things."

—*A spouse*

Nearly a third of all U.S. households have at least one person who served as an unpaid family caregiver within the last 12 months. More than 65 million individuals in the U.S. served as unpaid family caregivers to an adult or a child. That percentage of the population does not appear to have changed in recent years.

—*Caregiving in the U.S., a 2009 nationwide study by the non-profit National Alliance for Caregiving*

## Let's Get Your Spirit Ready for a New Day

Jot down the risks you have taken for love.

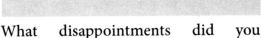

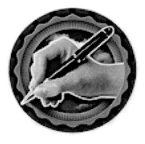

What disappointments did you experience?

# CHAPTER 5

# Weighing Costs and Promises

## My Voice...

Caregivers talk about their lives as both burdensome and rewarding. For many caregivers, life is a topsy-turvy blend of the two. Marriages have dissolved under the pressure; children can be unusually challenging; the air in a home can be filled with angry expletives; personal finances can crash until 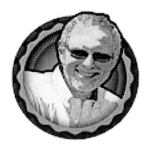 even the family home is lost. Those are only a few of the possible costs.

On the positive side, many caregivers report that they have never felt so personally needed and useful in their lives; marriages can grow stronger; children can be a source of hope and encouragement; the air in a home can be filled with laughter. Caregiving has opened doors to gifts people never knew they had.

Caregiving is an anvil on which is forged either strong or brittle steel.

# Wisdom of the Community...

"A mother chicken had two chicks.
One was well!
One was sick!
The mother chicken made chicken soup from the well chick to feed the sick chick!"

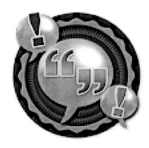

*—traditional parable*

"Sometimes I felt like I was achieving—or trying to achieve—for two people because there were things my sister, who is physically and intellectually disabled, was never going to do. I'm not sure if I felt that by myself or that it was a hybrid product of some of my mom's feelings too. I do think my mom was conflicted too—both about what sister would or would not do, as well as trying to overcompensate with me.

"I also don't know if I have an actual memory of this specific incident, or I remember it because my mom told it a number of times. I definitely know it goes to the guilt my mom felt. Once, when I was probably 3 or 4 years old, my parents had called my sister's pediatrician and left a message with the answering service because she was having a particularly difficult day. They ended up having to rush her to the ER and in their panic, left me at home. The doctor called after they left and I apparently pushed a chair to the phone, answered, told the doctor what happened, hung up, and walked next door—a distance of about 20 feet—to the neighbors' house to hang out. When the doctor arrived at the ER, he looked at my parents and said, "I know exactly what's happened, I talked with her sister." At that point, my mom realized what they had done and came home for me only to find me safely next door. I'm not sure my mom ever forgave herself for doing that.

"Perhaps one of the many reasons that I am who I am today—Type A, organized, focused—is, to some extent, that I had to learn to achieve for two. I developed a sense of self-sufficiency early because my parents did have to devote more time to my sister. I did my own and my sister's laundry from a young age. I cleaned—and I mean cleaned—and reorganized my room a lot growing up. Perhaps the repetitive behavior was comforting to a child/teen who had the medical unpredictability of a disabled sibling in her life."

*—A woman who grew up in a caregiving home*

"I am almost 30 and I have CP. My mother was my primary caregiver until I was almost 20. Then I moved out because living with my mother was like living in a box. My mother felt guilt and anger that she had me. She never understood my condition and her denial of reality was so strong that she thought someday I would wake up normal. School was my way out and I took it. I now live with my caregiver who understands and accepts me as I am."

*—A woman with cerebral palsy (CP)*

"The first few years that I cared for my husband were scary and uncertain times. I was always learning something new. When I finally accepted that he was lost to me—he would never be the man I loved and enjoyed—I surrendered. I accepted him as he was and I accepted me as someone who needed to learn from this and be a stronger person for the future. I opened some new doors and I have been opening new, exciting doors ever since. Caregiving saved and remade my life."

*—A wife*

"I have CP and I like to think I am independent because I know what I need. Actually, I still live with my mother, father and brother. They adopted me when I was one month old. I feel guilty that I have been such a burden. The adoption agency lied to them. They knew my condition and didn't inform my parents, but sent me anyway. My mother says she never regretted adopting me, but I feel guilt because I have been such a burden."

*—A woman with cerebral palsy (CP)*

---

"My child has come home and is living with me. He is 52. He is mentally ill and is not working. He is seeing a therapist and taking medication. I have no access to his therapist who says she can't talk with me because he won't give her permission. I don't know what and when he is to take his meds. He keeps me in the dark about a lot of stuff and if I complain he dismisses me as prying into his life. He tells me he wants my help, but I am kept on the outside. I think he is playing with me. I think about kicking him out and that feels like an awful choice. It is an awful situation, and I get more fearful and stressed each day."

*—A parent*

---

"It has just been all downhill for my son. He was such a gifted child in academics and sports. For some reason he got on drugs, then alcohol and now he has been in a hospital three times because of his mental condition. I'm so baffled and confused and angry and very guilty.
"I'm sure we failed him. I'm sure I failed him, but I don't know exactly how. I should have been a better parent—more responsive to his needs. I ought to have been there more for him. I'm sure he is a troubled soul because I have not been a good father."

*—A father*

---

"My mother has been in a nursing home for almost 4 years. She has a seizure disorder, Crohn's disease, and dementia. I go to see her every day. My whole life seems to be built around her. My dear husband had trigeminal neuralgia for about 3-4 years, had surgery on his trigeminal nerve (at the base of the brain) two years ago and has had a complete recovery. We are so blessed. He has never felt better. I retired from teaching about a year and a half ago, earlier than I had planned, but needed to take care of myself. There was just too much stress in my life. My grandchildren are the light of my life; two of them live here and two live close by in Austin. I try to spend as much time with them as possible."

*—A caregiver*

"Yes, I have clearly been through the caregiver wringer as well. It is very draining, very necessary, very difficult and very rewarding. It does focus our lives but not necessarily how we would like them to be focused."

*—A caregiver*

"Our marriage was destroyed. We lost respect for each other and had no common ground on how to deal with our son. Maybe it was just my husband's way of getting out of this family. He really couldn't cope with all of this. Now I do it on my own."

*—A wife and mother*

"A number of our old friends just drifted away. I never knew whether it was that they couldn't tolerate what was happening to us as this illness consumed our lives, or if we pulled back from them because we had no energy for a friendship. It meant we were more isolated. I give thanks for the friends who pushed to stay connected to us...it really helped in those really tough times."

*—A caregiver*

"We have three children, one with special needs. We both love her but we disagreed about so many things when it came to what was best for her. She is certainly not why our marriage failed, but I suspect she thinks she is. I'm sure the extra burdens we felt with her added the weight that brought our already shaky foundation down."

*—A parent*

"By the time my wife finally died I was totally depleted— emotionally, spiritually and physically. I rarely slept more than one hour at a time. I was constantly attending to her prescription schedule as well as to all the other details of her life and mine. Exhausted—absolutely *exhausted*!"

*—A husband*

"Burning resentment!!! I read once that 'resentment is a closet full of rusty swords.' I think I have been impaling myself on those rusty ol' swords too long. It's me that is suffering from my own resentment—not my siblings who have not helped out with the care of our father. I have been poisoning myself with the bile I feel toward them... not very smart, is it?"

*—A daughter*

Caregiving can range from a year to a lifetime. Overall, across the U.S., a third of caregivers say they've been providing services for less than a year, a third say it's been one to four years, and a third say it's been five years or more. At that point, long-term caregivers are significantly more likely to report a decline in their own health. At five years and beyond, 1 in 4 caregivers report a decline in their own health. Women are more likely than men to feel high levels of stress: 1 in 3 women vs. 1 in 4 men. Half of all caregivers say their choices have taken them away from friends and other family members. Those who have separated in this way are far more likely to feel high levels of stress.

> —*Caregiving in the U.S., a 2009 nationwide study by the non-profit National Alliance for Caregiving*

## Let's Get Your Spirit Ready for a New Day

What has caregiving cost you, your family?

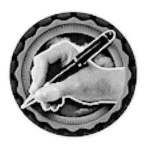

What are the promises you have reaped from caregiving?

# CHAPTER 6

# Appreciating Time, Fragile Time

## My Voice...

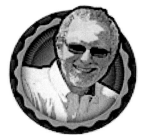

*Once upon a time,*
*Ordinary time became*
*Exceptional time—*
*Extreme time—*
*Fragile time.*
*Once beneath time,*
*When my soul slid beneath Presence*
*And I became too comfortable being*
*Alone,*
*I was fragile and brittle.*
*I might fall to pieces*
*Unless I can make the world go away!!*

Do you know the Greek mythology of Zeus's birth? His father, Cronus (the personification of chronological time), married his sister Rhea (who personified earth or ground, much like her better-known mother Gaia). As Rhea had children—Hestia, Demeter, Hera, Hades and Poseidon—Cronus was afraid of their potential power and devoured them immediately. To protect Zeus, her next child, Rhea hid him in a cave on Mt. Ida in Crete. Rhea substituted a stone wrapped like an infant for the hidden newborn and Cronus once again gulped it down. Eventually, Zeus emerged as a true threat to Cronus. Overthrowing

Cronus, Zeus forced him to belch up the stone along with the five siblings. Zeus now controlled what the world's great religions sought to control: time itself.

Caregivers understand that mythology. We understand that time eats us alive. Time can move so fast that it upends our world—or can drag along at an excruciatingly slow pace minute by minute, year after year.

This section of the book, "Telling Our Story," closes with this chapter on time because these two challenges are in a constant dance: honestly telling our story as it unfolds, and coping with the unpredictable time we have in this world. Avoidance of these truths is the keystone of emotional and spiritual anguish. Or, in a more colloquial form: It's what you avoid that will come around and bite your butt. For example, anger and the instinct to fight are among our natural protective defenses. But anger can often be a defense against facing our inner fears: loss of control, loss of a basic sense of personal identity—and loss of time.

In this book's opening pages, I told you that I will help you identify and also give you permission to feel, to think, to express a wide range of emotions, yearnings, fears and desires that are yours as a caregiver. In one way, this seems strange because we think we know our own feelings and don't think we need permission from anyone. Yet, the reality is that we can become so consumed by the tasks of caregiving, that we avoid expressing ourselves honestly. Often, we don't step back into our solitude long enough even to identify our true feelings. When anger, guilt, shame and fear crop up in our lives, they can be deeply disturbing—especially if we feel they are a contradiction of our compassion and empathy and the focus of our mission. These contradictory feelings, often surfacing at the same time, can leave us confused and stymied. In the end, we realize that we need permission to think, to feel and to express ourselves.

The poet James Truxell wrote "A Prayer from Far Away" shortly after Thanksgiving morning in 1998 to express the "absurd, undeserved pain" that can erupt in our lives when the daughter of dear friends left her home and crashed her car into a tree, killing her instantly. Her infant child survived. It is thought that she may have swerved to avoid a deer or possibly fallen asleep at the wheel. Afterward, Truxell said, "This poem-prayer was part of my response to this tragic event. It's a very, very raw prayer: honest, but raw." As you read Truxell's poem, may it inspire you to recall honest, raw responses to your own life now—even the confusing and tragic moments.

**A Prayer From Far Away**

*Sod!*
*I insist:*
*Do not yield so quickly to the*
*Grave digger's tool!*
*Not here! Not now!*
*Resist!*
*It is too soon for one so young*
*To be in your lonely, dark embrace.*
*I would deprive you,*
*Greedy earth,*
*Of this one from us so violently torn,*
*Like the shovel that now would part your roots.*

*God! I insist:*
*Yield quickly to my demand to know*
*By what rule?*
*Why her? Why now?*
*Desist!*
*It is too soon for one so young*
*To have "gone home to be with you."*
*I would deprive You,*
*Yes, You!*
*Would that I could with that shovel*
*Visit the back of your cosmic head!*

*Some small part of me –*
*The cerebrum, no doubt –*
*Knows that You aren't like that,*
*Not really:*
*Not one to snatch life away*
*Unfairly,*
*Absurdly,*
*Horribly.*

*Some small part of me—*
*A synapse or two—*
*Knows You are not a distant dictator—*
*Arbitrary and totalitarian in your decree—*
*Declaring "Take now this one;*
*And now the next!"*

*Some small part of me—*
*A molecule of serotonin dancing on a*
*Tiny, crowded floor—*
*Knows that You are among us as*
*One who also weeps,*
*Who knows the sting of*
*Wrongful death,*
*Absurd, undeserved pain;*
*As One who*
*Keeps the promise of*
*Being*
*Alongside of us in our tears,*
*As the One who will,*
*One more time,*
*Survive our rage and*
*Yet bring us all—*
*The dead and those of us who feel*
*We're dying—*
*Home.*

*But tonight the larger part of me, Lord,*
*Is far from home—*
*In a country far, far away—*
*Where now I ask to be handed the*
*Shovel.*
*Maybe I'll dig the grave myself,*
*Maybe lie down in it and take her place.*
*But maybe not,*
*For the larger part of me says this night:*
*"You'd better duck!"*

> —James M. Truxell, November 30, 1998

## Wisdom of the Community...

"I am so embarrassed—I told you four times I would write a couple of paragraphs for your book. I still haven't done it. I have it at the top of my to-do-list and every night when I notice it, I'm just so tired I collapse. I am so sorry. I shall try."

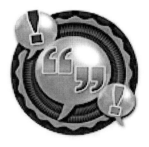

> —*A caregiver*

"I never seem to have a chance to rest!! I need just a pinch more time—there never seems to be enough!"

> —*A caregiver*

"I've spent most of my life waiting—always on hold. I don't get any real acknowledgment and appreciation for what I have done and been through from any members of my family."

> —*A caregiver*

"It's the way we caregivers live—like the crawl of a slug."

— *A caregiver*

"Time seems to drag when life feels so hard and then it rushes by when it seems like it is going well."

— *A caregiver*

*"Small things are magnified*
*With the shutting of the eyelids—*
*Too much imagination,*
*Anxiety,*
*Fear…*
*Where does my hope go when my eyelids shut?*
*Watching My Birds!*
*Birds on a wire—*
*From my watchtower—*
*I watch…I listen…I wait*
*In silence*
*For a Word…*
*Of comfort—hope—solace*
*A Dove…*
*Our Shrunken World*
*It is where we live now…*
*PAIN*
*Everyday, he is in pain*
*and I live,*
*endure,*
*grumpy moments—his and mine. "*

— *The poem of a caregiver*

"Waiting rooms are exhausting. How many times—how many hours have we spent in waiting rooms over the last ten years? Doctors' and Urgent Care Offices—they all look like cheap solutions to the problem of time—a way to keep the masses occupied and hopeful. Is there a waiting room anywhere with a current magazine?

"Yes, I get cynical, sometimes, very cynical—but underneath I go and wait and hope that this time we will get some decisive and permanent help. And, yes—once we get in there to the inner sanctum, nearly every nurse and every doctor does take us seriously, especially when we are there together."

*—A caregiver*

---

"Our world moves in slow motion—like molasses in January, as they used to say. There is no turtle and the hare race here, just turtles. That's us—slow and steady. We used to ride bicycles and herald the joys of seeing beautiful things we never saw while driving the car. Now we see beauty at an even slower pace—I walk next to him with his walker and we see what the turtle sees."

*—A caregiver*

---

## Let's Get Your Spirit Ready for a New Day

List two tasks you think that only *you* can do!

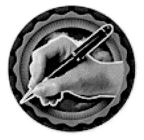

# Let's Imagine

Snow was not predicted during the night, but the half-inch dusting of snow has turned everything white and, of course, snarled traffic for commuters and for us, too. But it is especially beautiful in this early morning as the clouds clear and the sun glistens off the crystalline surface. We chat about the 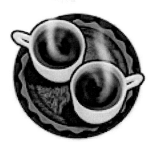 difficulties of arriving on time for our breakfast date—it is nothing new for either of us—we are always running off schedule.

This is becoming our place—toasted cinnamon bagel with honey, robust coffee, delicious, comforting and often confronting conversation.

At one point, after our pleasant small talk, I say, "The scariest, lowest moment in my life as a caregiver was the morning my wife mournfully said, 'We need to talk about the best time for me to kill myself. I can't—no—I won't continue to live in this daily pain and anguish.' I was stunned, scared, bewildered, uncertain of what to say or do. I knew it was bad—the depression was engulfing both of us, but I was not expecting this. It was the lowest point in our 43 years of marriage."

After a few minutes of silence you tell me about your most frightening, bewildering moment as a caregiver.

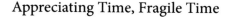

# PART 3
## Living in Community

# CHAPTER 7

# Finding Community

## My Voice...

This is a must: finding a community that will listen to you, sustain you and cradle you with care as you give care to your loved one. No, it is not easy. Yes, it takes time. No, it won't happen without your effort. Yes, I know that you can't imagine adding more to your already full agenda. Yet, it is a must!

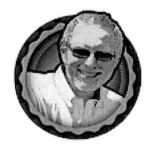

Here's a true parable of community—a story you may not have heard but that people remember vividly in the Special Olympics around Seattle. Some years ago, nine children lined up for the 100-yard dash, the gun went off, and these children began to move with relish down the line. Before they had gone even a third of the way, one child tripped and fell and skinned his knee, bloodied his hand and began to cry. By that time, all the other children were far ahead of him, but one by one they slowed, stopped and turned around. One little girl with Down's syndrome came back, knelt down and kissed his forehead and said, "This will make it feel better." The other children helped pull this child to his feet. All nine children locked arms and walked across the finish line together. Thousands of people shot to their feet and cheered long and hard.

Arm in arm, walking across the finish line together is an excellent metaphor for the kind of community that is invaluable when it comes to caregiving. It is a beautiful and necessary image of survival and contrasts vividly with doing the job alone.

In our American culture, the Lone Ranger has been a symbol of the individualism that many think made us a nation to be envied. We have the highest standard of living based on the vigor of our consumption, but not on the strength of our communal life. The loner who works for the good of others—with minimal reliance on companions—is an ideal permeating our national ethos. At the other extreme is the cry for community values that advocates the well being of all as the highest priority—sometimes over individual freedom. But neither extreme is a realistic answer. The value of the individual and the value of the community must be held in dialectic tension and both values must always be weighed carefully.

Caregivers and care receivers have a helpful phrase to describe the way they hope to build community: "entourage development." That's the process of forming a network to support our collective well being. The stronger the entourage, the more independent the caregiver and care receiver can remain. In this strategy, caregivers and care receivers are only as limited as the community allows.

## Wisdom of the Community...

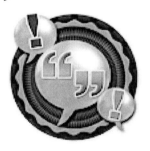

"Here is my best advice: make friends with senior citizens. Their loving care is invaluable. I suppose there are a number of ways that you can meet people in this category, but I have made these sorts of connections through my church community. One such person has taken it upon herself to see that every Sunday someone in our congregation spends a bit less than an hour with our daughter who is intellectually challenged. This effort on her part is probably the principle reason we have become regular attendees and been able to enjoy the many gifts a church community has to offer a young family. Well, we were young when we started. Someone else in the community, a single woman with grown children, approached me during a particularly difficult time when we were considering residential placement for our child. She had a connection at the school we were considering. She arranged a vacation day and drove me the five hour round trip to the school and offered me an introduction I would not have enjoyed otherwise. Another friend manages to contact me at least once a month for a luncheon / therapy session where he gently teases all my worries out of me. He asks questions and listens, truly listens, to all I have to say. I am forever flustered with the clock, but he always makes me feel like he is doing the most important thing in the world—hearing out his good friend. I've always thought that older people have a disproportionate amount of time to offer a binding friendship, but maybe it is just an earned wisdom that goes with their age. As I've aged, I certainly don't feel less busy."

*—A parent*

"My husband developed Alzheimer's and I got wonderful support from the community. My pastor said bluntly, 'Don't hide his condition—people know something is wrong. Fill in the blanks so they won't fill them in with false labels.' Then someone in my Sunday school class lined up twenty men who would be available to sit with my husband if and when I needed to get out. It saved my sanity. We had lived in the same community for many years—the neighbors were incredible. When my husband took the dog for a walk in the early years of his illness, all the neighbors kept an eye on him and helped him get back home if he got confused."

*—A wife*

"Because of our son's special needs (physical and mental limitations), he attended special education pre-school beginning at age three. Having our families nearby provided an immediate support system. We were lucky! Fortunately, before his birth I had decided to stay at home and put my career on the back burner. Some things are meant to be—since I was clearly needed at home.

"Five years later when his sister arrived, it was abundantly clear that extra hands would be needed to care for two children with very different requirements. Enter: an 'angel' or a 'gift from Heaven' as we are fond of saying! It was almost like a miracle that she was sent our way. She needed a job, even though she came equipped with two college degrees! Clearly, over-qualified for the job of providing extra hands, she nevertheless started her caregiver duties the very next day!

"I knew then, but also especially now (18 years later) that having the 'angel' available helped me keep my sanity as I juggled our son's ever-changing needs and the demands of my newborn daughter. I have often credited my husband with the wisdom (and generosity) to realize that by having help at home he knew it kept me sane and allowed my life to be more balanced. And, at the end of each day there was something left of me to enjoy time with my husband. I was able to keep my head above water and feel less defeated by each day's daunting challenges."

*—A parent*

---

"It's a funny thing about death. Sometimes, out of sadness, sorrow, and grief can come amazing, uplifting, and supportive acts of kindness. This is the story of how that happened to my family. Though our daughter-in-law had converted to our faith, Judaism, she felt that she wanted to return to her original upbringing in the Presbyterian Church, after her son was born. When he was 4 years old, they moved about 400 miles away, leaving a huge hole in our hearts and lives. I was adamant that I wanted to be a part of my grandson's life, and if that included attending his church, then that is what I would do when I was visiting. That turned out to be a very fortuitous decision.

"When our grandson was 9 years old his mother died. She died on her birthday. Our family was shaken to its core. One important piece of this story concerns our son who has severe learning disabilities. We could not begin to think how he could care for himself and a nine year old. He is a hard worker and gets minimum hourly pay but he is not capable of managing the money he earns or the money we provide. He primarily watches TV when he is not working and has little skill at providing basic care for his very bright son.

"Everyone in the church embraced our grandson—and his extended family. I began a long distance living arrangement, traveling back and forth between North Carolina and Virginia. In addition to filling their refrigerator and making sure bills were being paid, I began attending church with my grandson. I was, and am, warmly embraced and welcomed whenever I visit—members vie to tell me wonderful stories about him.

"I remember telling our grandson there was good and bad news about the little house we had just purchased for him and his father. The bad news was that there were no kids for him to play with. The good news was that he would have an abundance of grandparents! We met the neighbor living behind their house, a single woman, who was a retired government worker from our area in Northern Virginia. In the game of 'Six Degrees of Separation' we discovered that we had several friends in common. It was love at first sight. She embraced our entire family, and our grandson found a true and loving mentor. A more generous and caring person I cannot imagine. Our success in helping our son and grandson live on their own is due in no small measure to the assistance they receive from her.

She takes him to dental and orthodontia appointments; makes sure that he has rides to and from school activities; sees that he gets to his summer activities once school is out in June; embraces his love of jazz and often takes him to local concerts. This brings us full circle back to his Presbyterian Church. She is Catholic and attends mass at her church. She has a friend who was looking for a Presbyterian church to join. When I was in town the next time, I (the Jewish grandmother) took the friend to church and introduced her to my friends at the Presbyterian Church. She was warmly welcomed. Friends tease me by asking if I've done any recruiting for the Presbyterians lately.

"The list of neighbors who have helped in countless ways is remarkable. This past Mother's Day I sent cards to four women, thanking them again for being in our lives and helping us to care for our son and grandson. I can't imagine a more caring or supportive village!

"Two years after our daughter-in-law died we made arrangements to bury her ashes. I told my grandson that I didn't want to have a minister. I wanted us to conduct our own service. That was fine with him. 'When I grow up I'm going to be a part time minister!' he told me. 'What will you do the other part time?' I asked. 'I'm going to be a writer,' he answered. 'Ah, I see. Well I'm going to write a book too,' I replied. 'My book will be about how a Jewish grandmother raised a Presbyterian minister!'"

*—A parent and long-distance caregiver*

"Alone we can do so little; together we can do so much."

*—Helen Keller*

## Let's Get Your Spirit Ready for a New Day

Describe the community or communities that support you as a caregiver.

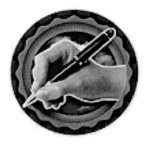

Whom do you trust enough to tell your story?

To whom do you reach out when you trip and fall?

If you suddenly find yourself in trouble, who is the first person you call? A friend? A co-worker? A relative? A neighbor? Someone in a local congregation or community group? Make a list and think about the nature of these relationships. How did they form?

Jot a few notes about a time when you reached out and someone helped to pull you to your feet again.

# CHAPTER 8

# Joining Support Groups

## My Voice...

Support groups can be a gateway to community and today they come in many forms. You may find such groups through churches, hospitals, libraries and local service organizations. City, county, state and national agencies also guide people to support groups. Advocacy networks now focus on a huge 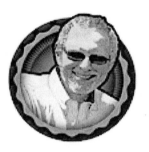 range of physical and mental challenges—and may recommend local support groups as well. The best groups are eager to help new families connect with experienced families, which can build healthy community. Some examples are listed on the website [www.GuideForCaregivers.info].

Support groups have long offered companionship and information for people coping with diseases, disabilities or caregiving. These groups generally provide vital forms of nonprofessional and nonmaterial aid: offering and evaluating relevant information; sharing personal experiences; listening to and accepting others' experiences; providing sympathetic understanding; and establishing social networks. Some groups work to inform the public or engage in advocacy. Some groups share physical resources—from reusing wheelchairs to providing expertise in building access ramps.

Most importantly, support groups maintain interpersonal contact among their members—meeting regularly and giving everyone an opportunity to talk. Health care professionals manage some support groups but the majority are focused on self-help and are managed by members who are commonly volunteers and have personal experience to share. These self-help groups may also be referred to as fellowships, peer support groups, lay organizations, mutual help or mutual aid groups.

Ask around your town about the range of support groups available. You may not like one group's format, but may discover that a second group is ideal. Membership in some support groups is formally controlled with admission requirements and membership fees. Other groups are "open" and allow anyone to attend advertised meetings or to participate in an online forum.

The Internet has provided an important new venue for support groups, but here's a word of caution: It is not difficult to find a local or an online support group, but it may be difficult to find a good one. Some online groups are run by pharmaceutical or medical-supply companies promoting a particular product. Some websites are not properly moderated and can turn into a Wild West of interactions. The website for this book [www.GuideForCaregivers.info] is not intended as a support group, but we are providing that safe space online for caregivers to post ideas, responses, reflections and questions as they work their way through this book. Our website is independently moderated and secure.

Before committing to any support group, see how it feels to you and ask local people you trust for advice: doctors, pastors, teachers, therapists—even local newspaper websites often list trusted groups.

# Wisdom of the Community...

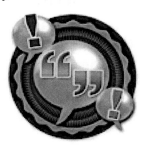

"I have had wonderful experiences and valuable help from my support group. I can't say enough good things about the group. I know a couple of people who have not had such positive experiences, but for me it has been good. One of the most valuable resources offered by my support group are the suggestions I have received about who are the good professional caregivers, doctors and therapists. Good doctors know how to listen to family caregivers. We are the ones who know the true situation. My support group has directed me to the doctors and therapists who not only treat my loved one very well, but treat me with concern and respect. They consider me part of the team."

*—A caregiver*

"I spend much of my life in a wheelchair because of CP. What I have and what I am able to do is a God-given gift. I have turned to religion because it nurtures me. I feed off the positive energy of the community in my church. I don't do very well on my own."

*—A woman living with cerebral palsy (CP)*

"I am for people. I can't help it."

*—Charlie Chaplin*

"If I can stop one heart from breaking,
I shall not live in vain;
If I can ease one life the aching,
Or cool one pain,
Or help one fainting robin
Unto his nest again,
I shall not live in vain."

—*Emily Dickinson*

---

"In the 1930s, Bill Wilson—known to millions as 'Bill W.'—described Utopia this way: 'We have it with us right here and now. Each day my friend's simple talk in our kitchen multiplies itself in a widening circle of peace on earth and good will to men.'

"He was drawing on a lively stream of American can-do teaching about health. In the 1800s, books by Clara Barton and Florence Nightingale urged all Americans to take health and recovery seriously. They taught men—and especially women, who formed the backbone of most American households at the time—to realize that illness and disability were not acts of God to be passively accepted. Barton and Nightingale felt that everyone should learn more about proper health care and responses to public-health issues.

"In the midst of the Great Depression, Bill W., Dr. Bob Smith and a small group of their friends tried an often painful experiment with their own lives. Eventually, they took the idea of self-help networks to a radical extreme and launched Alcoholics Anonymous. Their Twelve Step approach, drawing on a generic faith and the strength of mutual support, revolutionized both health care and organized religion, historians now acknowledge. In the

21st century, a vast network of support groups for every one of life's challenges now circles the globe."

> —*David Crumm, Editor of ReadTheSpirit online magazine*

## Let's Get Your Spirit Ready for a New Day

Are you aligned with a support group? Is it helpful?

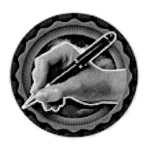

Name what you specifically want or need from a group.

What do you wish a support group would provide?

Are you aligned with an advocacy group? Name specific ways this has been helpful or not helpful.

Do you receive assistance from a service of your city, county or state?

What advice do you have for others seeking a support group?

Please share your experience with others through our website [www.GuideForCaregivers.info] .

# CHAPTER 9

# Savoring Solitude

## My Voice...

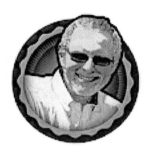

An essential counterbalance to our work as caregivers and our time within community is solitude. In the English language there are two words that express the condition of being alone. Loneliness frames the negative experience—isolating, divisive, and often painful. Solitude expresses the positive—self-connected, creative, rejuvenating.

Solitude can be found in many forms: meditating on a flower; basking in a sunset or sunrise; dancing alone in the rain; reading a good book; writing in a diary or journal; relaxing in a warm, soaking bath with candles and soft music; taking long walks in a forest or grassy field. The list is endless and the choice is individual.

Solitude restores us emotionally, spiritually and physically to face the rest of our lives.

## Wisdom of the Community...

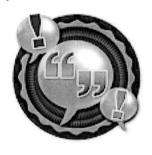

"I know that requests for solitude can be misinterpreted by those around us despite their love for us. I have had to make it clear in this caregiver journey more times than I can count that if I don't find time alone with myself I will fall apart. Many times a guest bath has offered itself as a retreat. It is amazing how comfortable a hard floor can be when you have to be alone with yourself and God on the 'Guest Bath Floor Retreat!'"

—*A caregiver*

"I'd like to get away from earth awhile
And then come back to it and begin over."

—*Robert Frost*

"Someplace where there isn't any trouble—do you suppose there is such a place, Toto? There must be. It's not a place you can get to by a boat or a train."

—*Dorothy in the Wizard of Oz*

"Very early in the morning, Jesus got up, went outside and walked to a solitary place to pray."

—*Mark 1:35*

"An early morning walk is a blessing for the whole day."

—*Henry David Thoreau*

## Let's Get Your Spirit Ready for a New Day

When and how do you most feel loneliness—that painful experience of being alone?

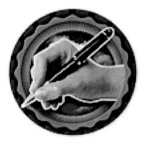

When and how do you experience solitude—that self-connected, creative, life giving side of being alone?

I invite you to do some exercises which might not be part of your normal routine. Here is one that may feel slightly uncomfortable at first, whether you do it alone or in a group setting. Take the risk. It can be revealing.

Do you remember the game we played as children in which we were twirled around and someone shouted, "Freeze!"? In my childhood it was called "statue." Picture in your mind's eye and then express them in statue form: your loneliness, then your solitude. Try it! Go ahead. What did you find?

Can you dance the two experiences? I bet you can. No one is watching.

# CHAPTER 10

# Admitting We Can't Do It Alone

## My Voice...

I don't need Sgt. Pepper to tell me that being a caregiver meets the entrance requirement to be a member of the Lonely Hearts Club. Too often, I thought I could do the job alone. It was a good way to become a hermit in my own home. I hunkered down and gritted my teeth and refused to let others do anything for me. I steeled myself in the beliefs and actions 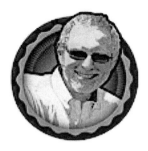 that I could do it by myself. That steel became the bars of a small prison that kept me in—and others who loved me, out.

Oh, I could make it on my own! Yet, I have learned that I couldn't become a genuine human on my own.

What keeps us from asking for help? Fear and pride, I suspect, are the basic reasons. Fear of giving up control, losing command of our own emotions, becoming inadequate and appearing less strong than we think we ought to be. Pride—especially in the form of being too proud for care—cripples our ability to invite others to share our burdens and joys.

We experience our task as daunting, and our challenges as ones that only *we* can shoulder. Often we receive little help, even from other members of the family. The very touchstones that define our lives—careers, loving relationships, friendships, even dreams—are sacrificed. If we share this reality with others, we open the door to those nearly overwhelming emotions.

But, let's turn the question around. How would you respond if someone asked you for help? Or more accurately and realistically, "What did you do when life asked you to respond as a caregiver?"

You answered, "Yes." You did not say, "Do it on your own—alone." So, live congruently! Don't let your own fear and pride keep you from asking someone else to help.

I realize that this admonition may seem naïve, unrealistic or even cruel in the face of the hard-core reality of your life. A grandmother who cares full time for her autistic grandchild must take rushed showers while her granddaughter is perched on the toilet. She has to constantly peer around the corner of the shower curtain to see that her granddaughter is not experiencing difficulty. I know that this is the reality of many caregivers who live every minute of their lives on the job.

Nevertheless, when our goal is the care of you—the caregivers—I must urge you to avoid the isolation that leads to loneliness and exhaustion. Millions of caregivers head down this road every year. The desire to reach out for assistance is not a sign of weakness—it is merely an indication of need!

Don't do the job alone! We are tackling a very tough issue here, so I want to counter with a lighter note. It has been many years since I came across the following letter to an insurance company. I have no idea who wrote it—all searches reveal the author is unknown. I have read it in various iterations and I have even heard a version sung by an Irish band. In spite of its humorous tone, I hope you will enjoy the funny side and ponder the poignancy.

# Wisdom of the Community...

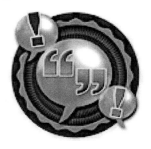

"Dear Sir:

I am writing in response to your request for more information concerning Block #11 on the insurance form which asks for 'the cause of injuries' wherein I put 'trying to do the job alone.' You said you needed more information so I trust the following will be sufficient.

"I am a brick layer by trade and on the date of injuries I was working alone laying brick around the top of a four story building when I realized that I had about five hundred pounds of brick left over. Rather than carry the brick down by hand, I decided to put them into a barrel and lower them by a pulley which was fastened to the top of the building. I secured the end of the rope at ground level and went up to the top of the building and loaded the bricks into the barrel and flung the barrel out with the bricks in it. I then went down and untied the rope holding it securely to insure the slow descent of the barrel.

"As you will note on block #6 of the insurance form, I weigh a hundred and forty-five pounds. Due to my shock at being jerked off the ground so swiftly, I lost my presence of mind and forgot to let go of the rope. Between the second and third floors I met the barrel coming down. This accounts for the bruises and lacerations on my upper body. Regaining my presence of mind, again I held tightly to the rope and proceeded rapidly up the side of the building not stopping until my right hand jammed in the pulley. This accounts for my broken thumb.

"Despite the pain, I retained my presence of mind and held tightly to the rope. At approximately the same time, however, the barrel of bricks hit the ground and the bottom fell out of the barrel. Devoid of the weight of the bricks, the barrel now weighed about fifty pounds. I again refer you to Block #6 and my weight.

"As you would guess, I began a rapid descent. In the vicinity of the second floor I met the barrel coming up. This explains the injuries to my legs and lower body. Slowed only slightly, I continued my descent landing on the pile of bricks. Fortunately my back was only sprained and the internal injuries were minimal. I am sorry to report, that at this point I again lost my presence of mind and let go of the rope. As you can imagine the empty barrel crashed down on me.

"I trust this answers your concern. Please know that I am finished 'trying to do the job alone.'
Sincerely yours."

> —*Anonymous*

---

"I don't really know who to turn to…I'm the one who has to get it done."

> —*A caregiver*

---

"It has become my job and my job alone. I can't burden others with my job."

> —*A caregiver*

---

"Yes, I'm a caregiver. I have always thought of that as a function of being a Christian pastor—a minister of the Good News. But lately I have been humbled by being the personal caregiver of a son who is intellectually strong but socially and emotionally, nearly disabled. My beliefs told me I was to be a sacrificial caregiver and if I was faithful I would need nothing else. Truth is—I was arrogantly stupid. I was too proud or too ashamed for care. I didn't reach out for help—I bore the burdens pridefully alone. You know, even Jesus didn't do that. Since I didn't take care of myself I ended up not giving my son the real care he needed."

*—A father*

---

"The most terrible poverty is loneliness and the feeling of being unloved."

*—Mother Teresa*

---

## Let's Get Your Spirit Ready for a New Day

Do you often feel that you can do the job alone?

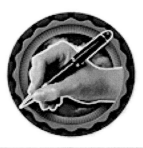

List a few of the reasons you give your-self when you decline to reach out for help.

List two tasks you think that only *you* can do!

### Look at these lists and ask yourself:

Are you still positive about those responses?

Now, name two people you have reached out to for assistance

recently.

What was your experience in reaching out?

**Name one person who gives you the most assistance with:**

Physical chores

Comfort

Peace and balance

# Let's Imagine

I didn't pay much attention to the weather this morning, but the excessive traffic did preoccupy me. It made me more anxious than I already was, because at every turn I was slowed down. I was eager, with a sense of urgency, to get to our meeting. Something compelled me to be with you at 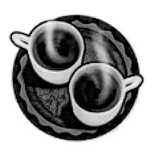 our familiar haunt, with bagels and coffee and your listening ear. I was needy, a state I don't admit to or accept often. Being with you is a much needed balm—an oasis of sanity and comfort.

After a quick greeting, I said: "I have two art pieces in my basement study which remind me of my yearning this morning.

One is a small 7-inch statue of a father embracing a prodigal son, a replica of the powerful symbol of forgiveness and compassion that stands in the gardens of the National Cathedral in Washington, D.C. The second piece, a photograph by Al Chang, is the image of a U.S. infantryman being comforted by a comrade as he mourns the death of a friend during the Korean War. In both pieces of art, one man is tenderly comforting another. I almost always identify with the comforter. With my size and my disposition, I have always assumed that position. During these recent days, I have wanted to be the one who is comforted."

**There is a brief pause and then you say:**

# PART 4

## Rediscovering Joy through Practices for the Body

# CHAPTER 11

# Paying Attention to Your Body

## My Voice...

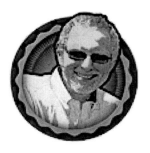

As a caregiver, how do you take care of your own body? Do you get a physical assessment regularly? Do you eat well, exercise regularly and rest adequately? Caregiving is demanding, stressful and time consuming. No one needs to tell you that. You also know that saying, "It's too hard," is never an acceptable excuse.

I am not going to make long lists of the foods you should eat or the exercises you should perform. You've got an ocean of that advice at your fingertips. I will say that most diets and most exercise regimens fail because we set impossible goals. Don't make a whole bunch of resolutions with the idea that you'll stick to them for the whole year. Instead, set goals for only two weeks at a time. Keep it simple. At the end of two weeks, assess your successes and your slip-ups. Be tender with yourself and then set goals for the next two weeks.

Start simple. Don't charge down the pathway toward physical fitness by purchasing a room full of exercise equipment. Start with a daily walk. Don't map out a diet for the rest of the year. Start with simple steps: Drink one glass of water before every meal or snack, or have a sweet or salty snack only after you eat a piece of fresh fruit first. You'll find long lists of such simple steps online, in your local library or physician's office.

The point is: Pay attention to your body! Take a few steps that can become a regular discipline. That's what a group of miners in Chile discovered when they were trapped underground for many days. They gave each person simple responsibilities for their survival which became a daily discipline. The miners survived together.

We all need good food, good exercise, an annual physical exam, time off from our caregiver duties. We need to know our own personal limitations. Our heads may lie to us—our bodies will not.

## Wisdom of the Community...

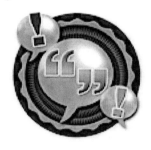

"I like comfort food—it tastes so good and soothes my aching heart. I like ice cream, mashed potatoes and gravy, salty chips and meat loaf. You wonder why I'm overweight and look ten years older than I am? It's simple. I turn to food for comfort when I am stressed. I turn to the refrigerator to comfort an ache in the pit of my stomach. I know some caregivers who turn to alcohol. Not me! I just turn to good ol' carbs to calm my stress."

—*A caregiver*

"My son's condition absorbs my time and my life. The one thing I do for myself 4 or 5 times a week is workout at the gym. I escape by furiously riding a bicycle for 50 minutes in a spinning class. I get very good exercise, and I may save my life and my sanity."

—*A caregiver*

"Somebody told me that I must never forget that caregiving is just one part of my life. She also told me that, 'So what!' needs to be part of my hourly vocabulary: 'So what if they sleep in their pants!' or 'So what if the floor is dirty!' Perfection and caregiving don't mix. Tea anyone?"

—*A caregiver*

"A healthy body is the guest chamber of the soul; a sick, its prison."

—*Francis Bacon*

"Exercise and application produce order in our affairs, health of body, cheerfulness of mind, and these make us precious to our friends."

—*Thomas Jefferson*

"Put your muscle where your mouth is."

—*Jack LaLanne*

# Let's Imagine

We meet again at the same café. You have invited me to breakfast, which feels very good to me. It's much cooler than when we last met, but still pleasant sitting out in the fresh air.

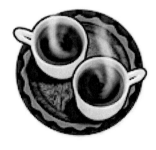

After sharing small talk, I say, "I have been following the story of the trapped Chilean miners. It fascinates me. I think they are offering a wonderful lesson to the world and especially to us caregivers. One lesson is the value of a disciplined daily schedule for coping with stressful situations. Each day in the mine begins just like a shift at 7:30 a.m. Each man has specific tasks under the direction of three group leaders who report to the managing foreman. Discipline is the order of each day. Breakfast is followed by morning showers under a natural waterfall located 300 yards up the tunnel. Morning chores follow. The men clean their living area. They have created a designated bathroom area and garbage area. They even separate recyclable materials. They care for their environment.

"The shift work is about basic sustenance—food, personal hygiene, maintenance of their environment and maintenance of their community through a general meeting following lunch, which always begins with group prayer. In addition, the men have an official pastor, an official group biographer and an official poet. It is the poet's verses of hope, gratitude and humor that have become some of the miners' most read messages around the world.

"The discipline helps the miners sustain their spirit and survive the ordeal. This is a great model for all of us living under stress!"

**You respond with thoughts about discipline and living under stress:**

# Appreciating Physical Presence

## My Voice...

People need more than words. They want our eyes and tears and smiles. They want our presence.

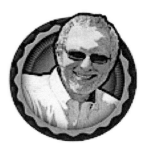

A mother sent her young daughter to the corner grocery for milk. When she didn't return as quickly as expected, the mother became concerned and went in search of her daughter. As she started down the street, the young girl was walking toward her.

The mother asked: "What took you so long? I was getting worried!"

The child responded: "When I was on my way to the store I met my friend whose kitten was killed in the street by a car. So I helped her."

"How did you help her?" asked the mother.

"I sat down with her and we cried together."

That's a tender and all-too-common story of one person entering into the pain of another. Have you ever cried with a friend who lost a pet, or got other bad news, or simply needed an attentive ear, a friendly face?

The great spiritual sages teach: Suffering doesn't need explanation—suffering needs personal presence. This is the origin of the Jewish custom of mourning known as *Shiva* —just sitting with family and friends for seven days. Other religious traditions encourage similar responses of presence.

Presence is the ability to be tender with another person. In making yourself available—or "present"—think of the tenderness of the girl in the story. There is an important difference between gentleness and tenderness. Gentleness is a kind action that respects the dignity of another and is a restraint of our own strength, but gentleness does not require self-revelation or a broken heart. Tenderness is born of intimacy and integrity in which you experience and share the vulnerability of the other person in the moment. Because tenderness always occurs in the context of mutual vulnerability, it usually precipitates a transformation of some kind. God's presence is experienced when we are tender—when we act as an instrument of God's healing presence by giving of ourselves—to listen, to love, to understand, to console—and to receive from another in return. People may not remember exactly what you did or what you said, but they will remember how you made them feel.

# Wisdom of the Community...

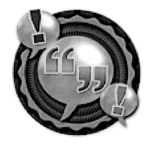

"A religious man is a person whose greatest passion is compassion."

—*Abraham Joshua Heschel*

"When death, the great Reconciler, has come, it is never our tenderness that we repent of, but our severity."

—*George Eliot*

"Ever'body might be just one big soul,
Well it looks that a-way to me."

—*Woodie Guthrie*

"A few months ago we were sitting at an outdoor café. The sky was very clear; the sun was comfortably warming our backs against the cool, brisk breeze of the early May morning; the coffee was very hot. I remember the hot coffee because it was while taking a cautious sip that her question chilled me to the bone. She had asked disturbing and probing questions before but this one struck especially deep.

"She is a friend I met a few years ago at an interfaith service project. We met as strangers and became friends working alongside each other. We've worked together occasionally through the years and meet for coffee to discuss children, grandchildren, politics and religion. She has been a sacrificial giver to her children and grandchildren. She is a devoted member of her synagogue and a spirited activist for social justice issues in her community. We share similar postures about politics and religion. Religiously, we both live out of the primary stories of our faith traditions that help to quiet our fears and sustain our hope and call us to be servants in the world. At least, that is the way we hope it is because neither of us sees religion as a set of beliefs but a way of being and doing in life.

"She has been quite ill this spring—so ill that she has feared that she might die soon. Her possible death is what we were beginning to discuss when I took the sip of hot coffee and she asked: 'Do you think I will go to hell?'

"Her question seemed so preposterous I quipped: 'Definitely, if you cause me to scald my mouth!' Then I looked at her and realized that she was serious. We stared at each other and then she said, 'I keep hearing on the radio and TV that I will go to hell unless I accept Jesus as my savior, which I am not going to do. Do you think I will go to hell?'

"I was stunned and then, to my surprise, I began to cry. I looked away. I just cried quietly and realized that the common view of hell and 'naming Jesus as my personal savior' has so pervaded our culture that it personally hurt a person of another faith tradition whom I deeply admire and love.

"I finally looked her in the eyes and said: 'No! No! I don't think you will go to hell—if there is such a place. I know you love and serve God faithfully. I—'

"She stopped me and said, 'Thank you—your tears already gave me the answer.' "

—*A truly compassionate friend*

---

"Yes, I feel helpless often! No, I can't do much about the big issues of our lives. I can do much about the small ones. I'm a caregiver, not a god or a doctor. As a caregiver, I can do something about some important issues—I can be present, listen, hold a hand, and give a cup of cool water. I am a caregiver—not a god!"

—*A caregiver*

---

"My wife and I were grocery shopping. She had the list and we were checking it twice. At one point, she said, 'I need olives,' and I responded that I would go find olives. I turned to go in the other direction from her to find olives when a nicely dressed older gentleman said, 'I need olives too.' Then, as we started walking together in the same direction, he said: 'You take good care of that woman, young man. My wife of 56 years died two weeks ago and I'm shopping here for the first time alone.'

"I said, 'Why don't we look for olives together.' Ten minutes later we still hadn't found the olives when my wife found us. But that didn't matter because I had learned all about his wonderful wife. He needed someone to listen and be present. I was the lucky one—he found me."

—*A caregiver*

---

"Life without a friend is death without a witness."
> —*A Spanish proverb*

"A faithful friend is a sturdy shelter; he who finds one finds a treasure.
A faithful friend is beyond price, no sum can balance his worth.
A faithful friend is a life-saving remedy."
> —*From Sirach 6 (or Ecclesiasticus)*

"Lord, make me an instrument of your peace. Where there is hatred, let me sow love. Where there is injury, pardon."
> —*Saint Francis of Assisi*

## Let's Get Your Spirit Ready for a New Day

Name two people who are present to you.

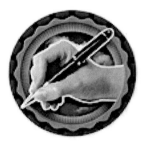

...to whom have you been present recently.

Do you have suggestions about being present that could help others? Please visit our website and share your thoughts [www.GuideForCaregiving.info] .

# Let's Imagine

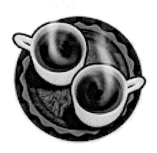

We have returned to the same bagel bakery and are enjoying cooler weather and a good, hot cup of coffee.

We share the pleasantries of seeing each other again and then I say: "I met with a chaplain friend of mine. She told me a startling story. A young Sudanese man, regarded as the spiritual leader for those in his village, found himself surrounded by the horror of gratuitous killing. In order to be less of a target to those bent on exterminating his tribe, nearly a thousand men, women and children would try to escape under the cover of darkness. They knew that, of the several groups that would begin the journey after sundown, at least one of them would be attacked and slaughtered during the night. The assaults were always from the air—impersonal and deadly.

"One morning, after such an attack on his group, he was surrounded by hundreds of dead and wounded villagers. The survivors came to him as their spiritual leader. When asked what he could possibly do in the face of such atrocity, his simple reply was that he would listen. He listened, because each of the survivors had to tell their story many times in order to find a way of coping with all that had happened: the attack, their survival and the death of loved ones and friends."

**You listen quietly even after I have spoken and then you respond...**

# CHAPTER 13

# Balancing Our Labor

## My Voice...

Throughout most of human history, manual labor was a natural part of life. Now, much of the work we do is intangible—mental, emotional, relational. All of the world's scriptures—as well as modern experts on fitness—teach that disciplined physical exertion is an essential part of healthy living. Call it 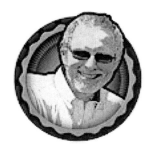 work, labor or physical exercise—we can't live without it.

We all know that in times of idleness or unemployment, we are more liable to succumb to depressive thoughts and feelings than when we are busy. (In the final section of this book, you'll find definitions of two forms of depressive conditions—burnout and accidie.) Regaining our health may take more than the intellectual or emotional connection we have with our current work. We may need to find intentional work that involves our whole physical being. I'm certainly not alone in offering this advice. It echoes through the millennia from spiritual sages to today's hottest corporate coaches.

You may want to skip this chapter! I realize that many of you already are fatigued from manual labor because the rigors of caregiving are often physically challenging. It is you, especially, who need the opposite of manual labor—you need the demands of mental, emotional and relational work. You'll find lots of ideas of such work throughout this book. To bring balance and restorative power to your life, you need to infuse it with disciplines of the mind and heart that are the opposite of your normal regimen. Balance is always the bottom line in sustaining or restoring our spirit. For millions of Americans today, however, manual labor is an unappreciated discipline.

A fascinating insight into this balance of labor comes from research by Michael J. Poulin, Ph.D. of the University of Buffalo, who shows that caregivers who actively participate in hands-on duties with their beloved will have less chance of slipping into depression than those who sit by in a passive posture waiting for some trouble to arise. So Poulin's advice to caregivers is: When someone offers to give you a break, invite them to come while your loved one is asleep or resting. Keep the hands-on moments for yourself.

## Wisdom of the Community...

"There is no substitute for hard work."

—*Thomas Edison*

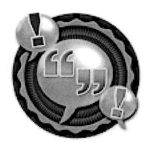

"I like to tinker with things. Sometimes I don't even wait for a problem. I tinker, I paint, I patch, I fix. It works for me. It keeps my mind active and my hands busy. Since I have become a caregiver I need these 'Fix-It-Up Chappie' tasks more than ever. It works for me."

—*A caregiver*

"My compost pile reminds me of my mortality. My aging, decaying flesh and bones will someday be scattered as ashes to nurture plants. I walk from my kitchen to the back corner of our lot and pour my vegetable scraps and coffee grounds on my compost pile. Then I take the garden fork and churn them in while I talk to the worms about their breakfast. Then in the spring, I sift the beautiful rich loam and gently feed my flowers. The whole process is like a sacred ritual that lifts my soul. It nourishes me to return to the house to care for my aging, decaying mother."

*—A caregiver*

"When I finish all the chores related to dressing, feeding and bathing my husband—getting him comfortable for a while—I go outside and play in my flower beds. I lose track of time and I never get hungry, even past lunchtime. If I don't get out there to play in the dirt, I want to eat all the time. I don't understand it, but I like being in my garden and not eating so much."

*—A wife*

"I once heard a preacher say that vacuuming could be a spiritual discipline. I thought he was crazy. I do all the vacuuming now that my wife can't do housework. Now I think that that ol' preacher may not be so crazy. This vacuuming has revealed to me how I have always looked for exciting, distracting activities to keep me from paying attention to my weakness, my mortality and my powerlessness. When I combine my vacuum learnings with what my wife's condition has shown me about my limitations, plus my ability to be gentle and present and caring—I have come to accept that you can teach an ol' dog some new tricks."

*—A caregiver*

"From labor there shall come forth rest."

*—Henry Wadsworth Longfellow*

## Let's Get Your Spirit Ready for a New Day

Which do you need more of right now? Manual labor? Relational labor?

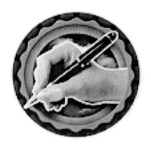

Now list 2 specific tasks that will possibly meet that need.

## Let's Imagine

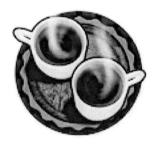

I've certainly come to enjoy these respite moments in this comfy, cozy, funky little bagel shop. I keep thinking of it as our place. It sends me back home with renewed energy for my tasks.

I say: "As much as I enjoy reading and being with friends, I have always needed time alone to do hard physical labor. The other day, I drove by a neighbor's pile of newly cut oak logs that were out for the trash. I don't even have a fireplace anymore, but I turned around and hefted ten or twelve of these huge pieces up into my little truck. I went home and moved them to the side of my house. Over the next couple of days I split those logs with great delight. I stacked them neatly and then later on I took them to a friend who loves his fireplace. May sound crazy, but that's me—a man who needs the pleasure of doing some hard labor."

**You make notes about manual labor in your life.**

# CHAPTER 14

# Singing

## My Voice...

How long has it been since you have burst forth in song? You don't have to do it when somebody's near. Just sing!

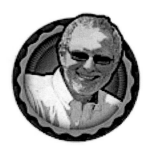

Singing is a sign that you probably are handling the stress of caregiving well. Or, it may be a way of reducing your stress and the tension that is held in your body and soul. Whether it's a tune from your prom or the first dance at your wedding, music is often associated with special memories and celebrations. Next time you listen to a song, notice how your body and mind respond. Are you swaying, tapping, or nodding your head and smiling? Music works the body. Music may reduce depression, anxiety, and the need for sedatives. Joyful music can lift your spirit and lessen your stress.

You may want to try what I have been doing for many years. When I go out in the morning to get the paper, whether it is 5:30 or 6:00 a.m., I sing a song of praise. It's about a 20-yard walk to the street where the paper is, and I don't care whether it's raining or snowing, or whether the sky is dark or beautiful with stars, I sing a song of thanksgiving. Some mornings I sing the Doxology, *Praise God From Whom all Blessings Flow.* Some mornings I sing the lively tune of gratitude that appears in the Albert Finney musical *Scrooge* . When Scrooge is taken by the Ghost of the Future to view the end of his life, he enters a street filled with people who are smiling, dancing and singing. Each singing person owed Mr. Scrooge a sizable amount of money. The debt was erased by his death. They sing as they dance around his coffin:

*"Thank you very much,*
*Thank you very much,*
*That's the nicest thing anyone's ever done for me..."*

No, I don't sing so loud that I wake my neighbors. But it is a way that I put a new and right spirit in me through singing. Music and singing have amazing restorative power in our lives. Like theater and art, music sends us soaring into new realms of the spirit while we are still grounded in our daily lives. When our daily lives are weighed down by onerous, exhausting tasks, music and dance can restore—even heal—something deep in our soul.

For those of you with a special affinity for religious music, I suggest you consider the following song. In the early 1600s, Martin Rinkart was a Lutheran pastor in a small town in Germany. The plague had spread throughout his community, and more than half his town and congregation was lost. He was conducting numerous funerals daily. In the midst of that loss, he wrote these startling words of faith:

*"Now thank we all our God, with heart and hands and voices,*
*Who wondrous things hath done, In whom his world rejoices;*
*Who, from our mothers' arms, Hath blessed us on our way*
*With countless gifts of love, And still is ours today."*

When your own spirit is broken, stressed, overwhelmed or bitter, this can be a very helpful verse to sing, read aloud, pray or meditate on quietly. It speaks of the God for whom many of us yearn. It defines the compassion we seek to offer to our loved one.

# WISDOM OF THE COMMUNITY...

"The day you open your mind to music, you're halfway to opening your mind to life."

—*Pete Townshend of The Who*

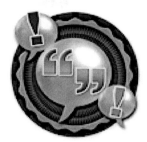

"I whistle a lot—whistle or hum— sometimes I don't even realize I'm doing it. It's not real loud and sometimes I realize I'm just doing it in my head. So, I guess you could just say that I whistle while I work. It keeps me going as I perform many of these less than pleasant, menial chores that come with this life of being a caregiver. My grandfather taught me to do it. He was a wildcat oil well driller in West Texas until the depression took his rig from him. When I lived with him, he was working as a gardener for rich families. He whistled a lot while he worked. He always said that it was difficult to get real sad and down if you whistled. A great gift he gave me—saves me on lots of days."

—*A caregiver*

"Yesterday, I needed a big dose of hope and a big kick in the butt. I was feeling a little too sluggish to do my tasks well. I needed a transfusion of joy. Suddenly, I started to whistle and then sing a little ditty. I was real surprised. I soon lifted myself out of the doldrums!"

—*A caregiver*

"I sometimes think the one thing that has enabled me to be a caregiver for so long is music. I always have music playing in the background. Sometimes I just stop and listen or sing along. It is a mini-break that refreshes me and centers, even restores me. I love music and what it does for me. I am so grateful for the people who wrote and play or sing and for those who invented radios and CDs. I can have music all the time. I think I wouldn't make it very well without my music."

—*A caregiver*

"I live my life in this wheelchair, but I love to laugh. I love to go to concerts and listen and move to the music, because it makes me smile inside. I listen to the radio a lot because I like music. I like to be in the hot tub with my caregiver because that's when I feel normal. We listen to music while we are warmed in the hot tub."

—*A person receiving care*

*"I sing a song of the saints of God,*
*Patient brave and true ...*
*They lived not only in ages past;*
*There are hundreds of thousands still.*
*The world is bright with the joyous saints*
*Who love to do Jesus' will.*
*You can meet them in school,*
*On the street, in the store,*
*In church, by the sea, in the house next door;*
*They are saints of God, whether rich or poor,*
*And I mean to be one too!"*

—*A popular hymn by Lesbia Scott, a busy mother with three children in 1920s England who loved singing so much that she wrote new songs to sing with her children.*

"Sweetest the strain when in the song, the singer has been lost."

—*Elizabeth Stuart Phelps*

"Music is the mediator between the spiritual and the sensual life."

—*Beethoven*

"He who sings scares away his woes."

—*Cervantes*

## Let's Get Your Spirit Ready for a New Day

**What kind of music makes you feel good?**

List some songs that lift your spirits—or a style of music—or an artist.

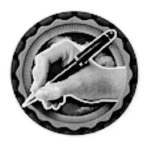

What inspires you to start singing, humming or whistling?

List some songs you enjoy singing.

Please consider adding your lists to our website [www.GuideForCaregiving.info] .

**Make your list a gift to someone else.**

Caregiving always involves grief and grieving. Try this exercise with music that might help you let go of some of your grief. You will need to select two pieces of music—the first is a piece of music that makes you feel most sad; the second is a piece of music that makes you feel most hopeful and joyous. These pieces can be long or short, vocal or instrumental—you choose.

Find a quiet place where you will not be interrupted. Close your eyes and begin to picture your loss. Play the piece of music you selected that makes you feel sad. Feel the music in your body in a way that expresses the depth of your loss. While you are listening to the music, you may discover that your hands are moving. If so, continue that movement.

When you have felt your grief, follow the same procedure but focus, this time, on the joyous music. Do you find yourself moving once again?

What selections did you play? Do you have a moment to share your experience to help others via our website [www. GuideForCaregiving.info] ?

# PART 5

## Rediscovering Joy through Practices for the Spirit

# CHAPTER 15

# Praying

## My Voice...

I am not big into prayer—at least when compared to others in my profession. Oh, I pray daily, but I pray on the run. I pray every time I hear a siren—it's a call to prayer and I pray for the afflicted and for the rescue workers. I seldom practice meditation, yet I am always processing in a meditative way.

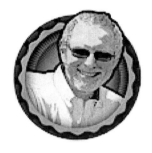

Every morning, I pray the Prayer of St. Francis to focus my actions (see below). That prayer grounds me and gives me direction. To pray it seriously is to know that I am never without a purpose and definition for my day. Persons of all faith traditions can pray it. This prayer calls me to claim my larger purpose in the midst of my mundane life. It calls me to be more than myself, to get beyond being sorry for myself. Helen Keller framed it well when she said: "Self-pity is our worst enemy and if we yield to it, we can never do anything wise in this world."

As I try to let St. Francis' prayer take hold in my life each day, my whole identity and sense of life's meaning is re-framed. The prayer reminds me that the world and my situation in life are no longer enemies—my circumstances no longer a cruel sentence. The prayer reclaims the world as a place where I live, work and serve with purpose and meaning. I am no longer passive. I am an active instrument seeking to make life less cruel. When I encounter hatred, injury, despair, doubt and sadness, my role is to sow seeds of love, pardon, hope and comfort. If I can allow myself to be made so, I shall be so—at least more often than not.

Many prayers can provide perspective for our lives. Holding them close to us can eventually transform our vision of each day and each small action we embrace as caregivers.

## Wisdom of the Community...

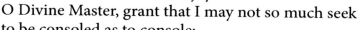

"Lord, make me an instrument of your peace.
Where there is hatred, let me sow love;
where there is injury, pardon;
where there is doubt, faith;
where there is despair, hope;
where there is darkness, light;
and where there is sadness, joy.
O Divine Master, grant that I may not so much seek
to be consoled as to console;
to be understood as to understand;
to be loved as to love.
For it is in giving that we receive;
it is in pardoning that we are pardoned;
and it is in dying that we are born to eternal life."

—*St. Francis of Assisi*

---

"I know that faith made my life possible and that of many others like me. ... Reason hardly warranted Anne Sullivan's attempt to transform a little half-human, half-animal, deaf-blind child into a complete human being. Neither science nor philosophy had set such a goal, but faith, the eye of love did. I did not know I had a soul. Then the God in a wise heart drew me out of nothingness with cords of human love and the life belt of language, and lo, I found myself. In my doubly shadowed world faith gives me a reason for trying to draw harmony out of a marred instrument. Faith is not a cushion for me to fall back upon; it is my working energy."

—*Helen Keller*

"There were actually 34 of us, because God never left us."

—*Jimmy Sanchez, 17, the youngest of the 33 Chilean miners who were trapped for over two months in the San Jose mine in Chile.*

"When I get to heaven, God is not going to be pleased with some of the things I have to say about the way life unfolds on this earth. I keep getting caught between a desire to quit and a very strong will to live. Being a caregiver is a blunt reminder of my own mortality and the mortality of the people I love. I know that I get philosophical—guess that is one of my coping skills. For example, I don't think I can be a person of faith without large doubts. Lately, being a caregiver has increased my doubts about God and this life. It has made me struggle to attempt to keep my faith in balance. The doubts weigh the most on this scale at present."

—*A caregiver*

"God, give us grace to accept with serenity
the things that cannot be changed,
Courage to change the things
which should be changed,
and the Wisdom to distinguish
the one from the other.
Living one day at a time,
Enjoying one moment at a time,
Accepting hardship as a pathway to peace,
Taking, as Jesus did,

This sinful world as it is,
Not as I would have it,
Trusting that You will make all things right,
If I surrender to Your will,
So that I may be reasonably happy in this life,
And supremely happy with You forever in the next."

—*The Serenity Prayer, credited to Reinhold Niebuhr (1892-1971)*

"Our Father who art in heaven,
Hallowed by thy name; thy Kingdom come;
Thy will be done on earth as it is in heaven.
Give us this day our daily bread.
And forgive us our trespasses, as we forgive those who trespass against us.
And lead us not into temptation, but deliver us from evil.
For thine is the kingdom, the power, and the glory, forever."

—*The Lord's Prayer*

## Let's Get Your Spirit Ready for a New Day

Do your actions, resulting from your faith, make any difference in your journey as a caregiver?

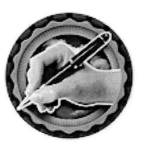

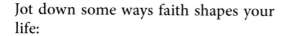

Jot down some ways faith shapes your life:

Prayer doesn't require a text. Prayer can arise spontaneously from within you. Many people start prayers with simple phrases, such as, "Open my eyes to …"
What situations inspire prayer in your life?

What prayers do you find helpful?

I've shared some of my own mainstay prayers above. Please share yours on our website [www.GuideForCaregiving.info] .

## Let's Imagine

Fall is definitely in the air—an early morning chill leaves us huddled in our fleece as we sit at a table outside, hoping the bright sun will soon warm us. We do like the outside setting.

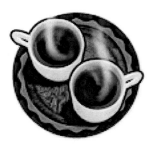

You ask if I believe in God and I answer: "Do I believe in God? Does my faith make any difference in this journey as a caregiver? I suppose the answer is yes. But for me, it is no longer the relevant question. I used to have fun arguing and struggling with theological questions that debate the existence of God. But that's not the really important struggle for me now. What is vital to me now is to act as if God exists in my daily life. Am I living as if God does exist as part of my journey—crying, laughing, loving with me along the way? Am I present to my beloved in a manner that portrays the way I long for an incarnational, caring God to be with us—present, laughing, weeping, often helpless, but benevolently attentive?

"So every day, often many times a day, I pray some portion of the pivotal prayer of discipleship, the Prayer of St. Francis. I yearn to act as if I, even I, can seek more to comfort than be comforted; to seek more to understand than to be understood and to seek more to love than to be loved. I know that I often falter and even fail, but singing songs that lift my spirit and praying prayers that remind me of this deep yearning often get me back on track as a giver rather than a brittle, laconic cynic. I try to live the answer rather than ask the question."

**You respond by answering the question: "Does my faith make a difference in this journey as a caregiver?"**

# CHAPTER 16

# Carrying Words with You

## My Voice...

"I have no time to read!" I've heard that from many caregivers and it's true in my own caregiving experience, but here's a practical tip that many have used over the centuries: Choose two or three very brief phrases and carry them with you! Of course, this is the same idea embodied in the prayer beads

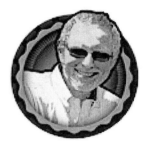

that are used in many traditions around the world—the beads become the reminders of phrases that men and women carry with them in their heads. But, I'm talking here about something even more tangible: Write helpful lines on scraps of paper and post them on the refrigerator door; hang them above the sink; scrawl them across the bathroom mirror!

For example, I know when my spouse is in a lot of pain. I can tell by her walk or the tone of her voice. I can see it in her eyes. On such a day, I might scribble, "Lord, make me an instrument of comfort to quiet the pain." I may place that simple yearning in my pocket. Each time I reach in, I am reminded of my focus. Or, I may write the phrase, "God, give us grace to accept with serenity the things that cannot be changed," and place it on the ledge above the kitchen sink. The notes jolt me into mindfulness and acceptance of our current reality as a couple.

You know what you need each day—what touches you, restores or lifts your spirit and keeps you focused. You may already have notes scattered throughout your home.

When I asked one caregiver to share her tips about carrying words, she sent back this note: "Boy, did your email take me for a journey this afternoon! I remembered verses that I always kept in mind every day as I cared for my husband throughout his nine-year decline with Alzheimer's!"

So, in the next section of this chapter, I've collected some words of wisdom that others have used in this way. Feel free to use them. I'm sure you'll discover more on your own, too!

# Wisdom of the Community...

"This too shall pass."

> —*Ancient aphorism*

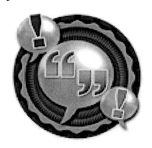

"All shall be well
And all shall be well
And all manner of things shall be well."

> —*Dame Julian of Norwich*

"I can do all things through him who strengthens me."

> —*Philippians 4:13*

"I long to accomplish a great and noble task, but it is my chief duty to accomplish small tasks as if they were great and noble."

> —*Helen Keller*

"You are not obligated to finish the task, but neither are you free to neglect it."

> —*Pirkei Avot 2:20-21*

"Life is short! Break the rules, kiss slowly, love truly, forgive quickly, laugh uncontrollably, and never regret anything that makes you smile."

*—Mark Twain*

"It is not the mountains that we conquer, but ourselves."

*—Sir Edmund Hillary*

"Neither a lofty degree of intelligence nor imagination nor both together go into the making of genius. Love, love, love, that is the soul of genius."

*—Wolfgang Amadeus Mozart*

"It's not the years in your life that count. It's the life in your years."

*—Abraham Lincoln*

"There are only two ways to live your life. One is as though nothing is a miracle. The other is as though everything is a miracle."

*—Albert Einstein*

"Wounds that can't be seen are more painful than those that can be seen and cured by a doctor."

*—Nelson Mandela*

"The question is not what you look at, but what you see."

*—Henry David Thoreau*

## Let's Get Your Spirit Ready for a New Day

Is there wisdom you carry with you every day?

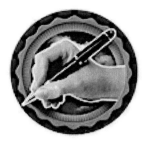

In what form do you keep it?

Do you use prayer beads or stones to hold your wisdom?

Jot down the basics of your practice:

Please consider sharing your wisdom and how you carry it with others on our website [www.GuideForCaregivers.info] .

# CHAPTER 17

# Journaling

## My Voice...

Are you keeping a journal? Some caregivers do and many do not. No particular rules are necessary except that it is important to keep it private unless you wish to share it with special people. A journal is a place for you to record your feelings, thoughts and even a daily log of your activities. Many find it help-

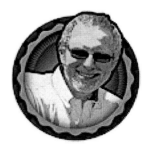

ful to record verses or snatches of wisdom from their readings. Some people write their feelings and thoughts in free verse. It is a way to capture a moment—a smell, a taste, a feeling, a joy or a sorrow.

A journal is for you. It is for you to craft in a way that best strengthens your soul and spirit. It is not something that is useful for everyone. For some, it just takes more time than you want or have because it is not what nurtures your soul. So, please make it useful to you—or scrap it.

## Wisdom of the Community...

"Recently, I decided to find my journal that I kept during the long years of my husband's decline. The journal starts on December 31, 2001 and ends on December 29, 2006. There are long dry spells and then lots of entries. I've spent the afternoon reliving a lot of memories. Funny,

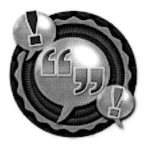

but I now see the journal differently than I did then. Then

I used it to just keep going but today I can see that I was also preparing myself for the future. The first entry in the journal is from *Man's Search for Meaning* by Vicktor E. Frankl: 'The last of human freedoms—the ability to choose one's attitude in a given set of circumstances' and 'saying yes to life in spite of everything.'"

*—A caregiver*

---

"I have lived much that I have not written, but I have written nothing that I have not lived."

*—Clara Barton, founder of the American Red Cross*

---

"Teach us to number our days that we may gain a heart of wisdom."

*—Psalm 90*

---

"I have come to believe that by and large the human family all has the same secrets, which are both very telling and very important to tell."

*—Frederic Buechner*

---

# Let's Get Your Spirit Ready for a New Day

Do you like to write? Is it something that comforts, calms, processes and records your thoughts and experiences?

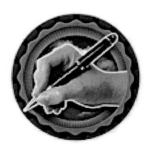

You are invited to share any advice you may have about journaling with other caregivers at our website [www. GuideForCaregivers.info] .

# CHAPTER 18

# Enjoying Poetry

## My Voice...

Have you discovered the power of poetry to inspire and sustain your spirit in difficult times? Thanks to Hollywood, the whole world knows that Nelson Mandela was inspired by the poem, *Invictus,* during his long imprisonment on Robben Island. He recited it and taught it to other prisoners. It

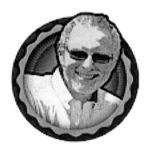

may well be that Mandela's inspiration came as much from the personal story of the poem's author as from its words. At the age of 12, William E. Henley fell victim to tuberculosis of the bone. A few years later the disease progressed to his foot. His life was saved by amputation directly below the knee. Despite his disability, he survived and led an active life until the age of fifty-three. The poem title, *Invictus,* is Latin for "unconquered." Certainly both men sustained an unconquered spirit through their challenge-filled lives.

Some poetry may make your eyes glaze over. Other poetry can make your soul dance, your heart resonate or your mind delight in the challenge. Poetry can put a name to feelings and emotions that otherwise elude us. Only you can know what speaks to your soul.

Listen.

# Wisdom of the Community...

### Invictus

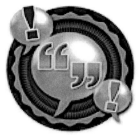

*"Out of the night that covers me,*
*Black as the pit from pole to pole,*
*I thank whatever gods may be*
*For my unconquerable soul.*
*In the fell clutch of circumstance*
*I have not winced nor cried aloud.*
*Under the bludgeonings of chance*
*My head is bloody, but unbowed.*
*Beyond this place of wrath and tears*
*Looms but the Horror of the shade,*
*And yet the menace of the years*
*Finds and shall find me unafraid.*
*It matters not how strait the gate,*
*How charged with punishments the scroll,*
*I am the master of my fate:*
*I am the captain of my soul."*

— *William Ernest Henley, 1849–1903*

"Words are always getting conventionalized to some secondary meaning. It is one of the works of poetry to take the truants in custody and bring them back to their right senses."

— *W.B. Yeats*

"Poetry is nothing but healthy speech."

— *Henry David Thoreau*

"A poem is a naked person."

— *Bob Dylan*

## Nuts

"Unless a seed fall to the ground and die, it cannot bring
forth new life."
—Jesus

*"Spring begins with a CRACK! of the bat*
*In a park with the cheers. . . .*
*Spring begins with a CRACK! in the heart*
*That breaks, spilling tears. . . .*
*Spring begins in the dark*
*Where there's no one who hears*
*The shell of the nut going CRACK!*
*Listen!*
*The green shoot appears!*
*Behind brown hardness since the Fall,*
*It waits. . .silently. . .darkly*
*And wishes for*
*All it's worth to be known. . .*
*Its secrets bare. . .*
*But not here! Not there!*
*Not now! It is too soon.*
*(The sun, at noon,*
*Yet is slanting low.)*
*And so, defended 'gainst the mortal cold,*
*Its own counsel keeps, and sleeps*
*Down within the humus*
*And the mold:*
*Where it is grateful for that structured, strictured,*
*Boundaried husk which*
*Gives not life,*
*Yet saves it by the purchase of some time:*
*Swaddling time. . .holding time. . .*
*Until, in time's fullness, ready,*
*It answers the subversive call of Spring*
*(That perverse Mystery of death and birth so mingling.)*

CRACK! the shell's embrace is broken free,
Releasing -- in giddy, adolescent mirth --
Into the damp and warming earth
A new, green wager that now the sun is right.

But what of that now-spent shell,
Whose broken, ugly shards repel
The notice of squirrels and
Other connoisseurs of Spring?
A funeral of dignity and celebration
Is its due.
So let the word go forth,
Sounded by the trumpets on the vine,
That it gave up its life in the fine
Service of protecting what it could not give:
Abundant liveliness to live!
Above let its marker be the green,
Rich extravagance that once was only dream
In silence and in secret.
And on that marker let its epitaph be read:
"I held on not too long, too tight,
But broke and bled,
To let the green life out. . .
Certain that the sun was right!"

　　　　—James Truxell

**Prayer Poem**

*"I NEVER saw a moor,*
*I never saw the sea;*
*Yet know I how the heather looks,*
*And what a wave must be.*
*I never spoke with God,*
*Nor visited in heaven;*
*Yet certain am I of the spot*
*As if the chart were given."*

      *—Emily Dickinson*

## Let's Get Your Spirit Ready for a New Day

Choose a favorite poem that speaks to your soul. Please write or print it out with pen or pencil. Don't type it—write it. Stand and recite it aloud in a private place. Consider reading it to your loved one. Writing in long hand and reciting a favorite poem can reduce stress and restore energy.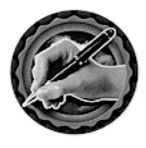

Also, don't hesitate to write your feelings and thoughts by composing your own poem. This, too, can reduce stress and restore energy.

Please share your favorite poem, as well as some you have written, with others at our Guide for Caregivers website [www.GuideForCaregivers.info]

# CHAPTER 19

# Grieving

## My Voice...

Caregivers live with loss and grief— a reality at the heart of the caregiver and care receiver relationship. Loss must be faced, focused and named so that we can grieve. After a major loss, only the grieving path can soften our dried heart, nurture us with humility and, in time, cradle gratitude in our souls.

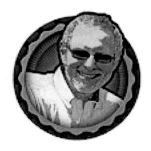

Grief is natural when someone who matters deeply to us is no longer accessible to us in the way we'd wish. Suddenly, our world is jumbled. A spouse, child or friend dies—or is diminished by a physical, mental or emotional disability. This grief can linger for years, especially when resurfaced by annual milestones of remembrance: holidays, visits to favorite places or even the return of that first spring day when the two of you loved to put the boat into the water each year.

Soon, we realize that dreams have vanished along with our loss. The dream of a stimulating marriage is replaced by the routine, mundane patter of caregiving. An occupational dream is squelched by financial stress. The loss of dreams is often not as obvious as physical loss, but their fading can drape a wet, gray blanket over life. Sometimes, it's difficult to discern that this is happening. We may grieve the loss of a spouse and ignore an equally deep need to mourn the loss of our dreams about that relationship.

Grieving is a primary spiritual practice that engages heart, mind and soul. Ultimately, grieving is the process of accepting the world as it comes to us, filled with limitations and possibilities; vulnerability and strength; love and hate; and winning and losing. It is the process of compassionately embracing the world again—as it is now. The more something or someone matters, the longer and harder we grieve. Some wounds never heal completely and leave us with a limp in our being.

Joy, hope, faith, trust and gratitude are gifts one receives along the journey of grieving. Hope and joy come on the heels of hard times, born out of the ashes of impotence. Faith comes as we accept what is ours in God's world. As we journey, we learn to trust and gratitude blossoms.

If we define grieving as facing the horror we have experienced and giving up the hope of a different past, then we are also describing key elements of forgiveness. The two are intertwined. Grieving may mean that we forgive God, forgive others—and forgive ourselves. As we mourn, we gradually let go of our imprisoning fixation on what has happened. By forgiving, we pave the way for joy and gratitude to return.

If we try to run away from the grieving process, we can find ourselves in two well-traveled lanes with potentially lethal ends. First is the high-speed lane of anger that can move toward rage. Speeding along this lane can result in violence, even homicide. The other extreme is the slow-speed lane of bitter resentment that gradually shuts down our mind, body and spirit. If unchecked, this lane moves deeply into accidie, the hopeless despair that could eventually lead to suicide. (See the "Resources" section at the end of this book for more on accidie.)

In all the world's great spiritual traditions, grieving is a life-giving discipline that leads us back to compassion and, ultimately, to joy.

# Wisdom of the Community...

"A light here required a shadow there."

　—*Virginia Woolf*

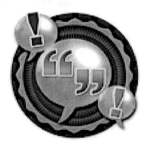

"A happy life consists not in the absence, but in the mastery of hardships."

　—*Helen Keller*

"I was determined to enter his world. I knew—I accepted—that he could not return to my world. Alzheimer's changed our world and separated us from our past and determined our future. I never asked 'Why God?' Here is a statement that I think helps explain my attitude. It's from *Your Sacred Self* by Wayne Dyer. A definition of enlightenment: 'the quiet acceptance of what is. I believe that truly enlightened beings are those who refuse to allow themselves to be distressed over things that simply are the way they are.'"

　—*A caregiver*

"Tears are the language I use when I don't have words—sometimes they are tears of joy or gratitude or hope. Other times, tears express my sadness that floods my weary heart and soul."

　—*A caregiver*

"Plans!?! The places we wanted to go until reality kicked us in the gut and changed our life course! They were our plans! Now, they are dreams that seem to have dried up like raisins in the sun. Our latest plan is to bake oatmeal raisin cookies. At least that will please our taste buds where we are!

"We were very frugal. We saved for a rainy day and for the day when we had all the money necessary to go to the places we dreamed of going without going into debt. I remember a story I read once about a woman who was given a very special small bar of soap. She put it in a drawer to use on a very special occasion. Years later, she discovered that bar of soap and was saddened that the time had never come to use it. She opened it and it had turned to powder."

*—A caregiver*

---

"Yesterday, my son's 45th birthday, ripped open the often so very fragile thread that holds my broken heart together even though that thread is the color of faith. I feel and love deeply and passionately and am one who likes to make things 'right,' whatever that is. 'Right' opens a whole new box. Who do I think I am to control God's creation? We celebrated his life yesterday by taking him on a long ride from Northern Virginia to the Skyline Drive. His sister packed a gift for him of favorite junk food items. My grief for him about what he cannot know and enjoy on this side of heaven is often triggered by expected or some not-expected moments. His birthday yesterday was one of them. Not until I was home did I allow myself to go to that painful place. I accept that, for me, grief is not a reality I will ever be without. The grief takes a better place when I affirm that God loves him more than me, and that he is first God's child, then mine. Only then can I be in the presence of God and His grace. Grief can be sometimes understood, given a place—but for me, grief will always be present."

*—A caregiver*

---

"Grief tears his heart, and drives him to and fro,

In all the raging impotence of woe."

> —*Homer, describing a father's grief over the loss of his son in the Iliad*

"Everyone can master a grief—but he who has it."

> —*William Shakespeare in Much Ado about Nothing*

"Believe me, it is no time for words when the wounds are fresh and bleeding; no time for homilies when the lightning's shaft has smitten. ... Then, let the comforter be silent; let him sustain by his presence, not by his preaching."

> —*The Rev. George C. Lorimer, advising comforters in 1881*

"Grief is the price we pay for love."

> —*Queen Elizabeth II after the terrorist attacks on 9/11/2001*

# Let's Get Your Spirit Ready for a New Day

**This whole book is filled with the necessary practices for grieving.**

Have you named with openness and honesty the "what is" in your life?

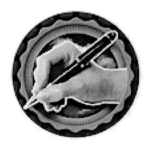

Without illusion, can you honestly

describe your life right now?

What are you grieving in this life?

Are you telling your story in a community you trust?

Are you living with presence, gratitude, music, art, humor and practices that sustain and balance your heart, mind and body?

When do you cry?

Where do you cry?

If you have helpful ideas about the journey of grief and recovery, please add a note to our website. [www.GuideFor-Caregivers.info] .

CHAPTER **20**

# Thanking

## My Voice...

Have you explored the previous chapter on grieving? That journey's destination can be gratitude. Perhaps real recovery takes place only when we take our wounded wisdom and turn it into generous gratitude to share with others.

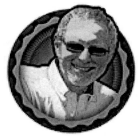

"I must love myself into action—lest I wither in despair," Alfred, Lord Tennyson declared after the death of a close friend.

These words sound so noble, but what are the first steps? Well, often they are physical steps—like pushing pedals on a bicycle. Sometimes, gratitude blossoms most fully in physical move-ment: Perhaps traveling to visit a friend; or, to another extreme, getting one's flabby body into training, then riding 400 miles to raise money for brothers and sisters afflicted with AIDS. I've talked to people who have fulfilled that challenge and every sin-gle one of them describes the deep healing they experienced in their own lives. The joy and gratitude they felt was exquisite!

In Europe, many pilgrims set out each year on the Way of St. James—a vast web of centuries-old routes that all lead to the Cathedral of Santiago de Compostela in Spain. Many are prayerfully seeking answers; most are walking with hearts brimming with gratitude.

There's a story about an elderly man crossing town on a city bus. His suit is a little too tight as he sits on the edge of his seat holding a bouquet of freshly cut flowers. He notices a little girl whose eyes are fixed on the flowers. Each time he looks, she is staring at his flowers. Finally he rises, hands the bouquet to her and says, "I cut these for my wife but she would want you to have them." She smiles. Then she watches him leave the bus and enter through the gate of a small cemetery.

"One" is the famous song by Bono and his band U2. Near the end of the chorus are these words: "We get to carry each other." When men and women around the world sing along, we're joining in a global hymn of gratitude. Life, then, is not about building bigger mansions, developing larger portfolios or praying sweetly or devoutly. It is about seeing the help that we give to others, not as a burden—but as a privilege. That is when gratitude becomes integral to the life of a caregiver. It is a true sign that our grieving has turned to thankfulness for the life we live.

## Wisdom of the Community...

"If you share your wealth sparingly, you will reap sparingly, but if you sow bountifully, you will reap bountifully."

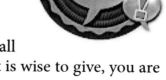

—*2 Corinthians 9:6*

"If you give freely you will grow all the richer; if you withhold what it is wise to give, you are likely to suffer want."

—*Proverbs 11:24*

"Whoever does not express his gratitude to people will never be grateful to God."

—*Prophet Muhammad*

*"I think God might be a little prejudiced.*
*For once He asked me to join Him*
*on a walk through this world,*
*and we gazed into every heart on this earth,*
*and I noticed He lingered a bit longer*
*before any face that was weeping,*
*and before any eyes that were laughing.*
*And sometimes when we passed*
*a soul in worship*
*God too would kneel down.*
*I have come to learn:*
*God adores His creation."*

> —*St. Francis of Assisi*

---

"If the only prayer you say in your life is 'Thank you'—that will suffice."

> —*Meister Eckhart, 13th Century*

---

"Thankfulness is the tune of angels."

> —*Edmund Spenser, 16th Century*

---

"The other day, I was examining all the prescription bottles in our cabinet. I suddenly felt grateful for the amazing miracles of modern medicine and chemistry. Then I thought: Maybe the most amazing miracle is that I stay present to my child with my love, my hope, my little comforting acts, my encouragement and even a regular smile. I let myself feel very good about what I do as a caregiver. We humans are small—finite—mortal—very vulnerable—capable of great atrocities and evil. But we are equally capable of magnificent acts of compassion and relational beauty. It is my time to show the latter to my beloved."

> —*A caregiving parent*

---

"I don't understand it. I don't understand it all. It is counter-intuitive but I have felt it. Many folks I have met and talked with about the process tell me that it is true for them. For some reason, if I let myself grieve—honestly grieve—that is, face the dream of who we were together, cry and moan and weep over the end of the dream—I let myself really experience the pain about my loss of my relationship with my spouse who has been enveloped by his illness—then I am released for a new sense of life and love. I relate to him differently. I stop wishing that he were someone else. I stop wishing he were not sick. I just accept the fact that this is the way he is and that we have a new relationship. When I reach that point, new windows and doors open. I feel lighter. The only way I can describe it is that I am filled with gratitude. Nothing objectively changes, but I change. I continue with my caregiving tasks but with a different heart. I start feeling joy when I least expect it. I find myself exclaiming gratitude for the smallest things— the beauty of a sunset, a flower, a meal brought by a friend and a multitude of other simple events."

*—A caregiver*

"I always seek to remember that I, who need community and uplifting, can still look for ways to be of use to others outside of my need. I watch for the moment to provide community and solace for others, to bring balance and joy into our world. I remember when we had volunteers come to our home seven days a week, eight hours a day. I would sit on the porch waiting for the next shift to come and I'd pray: 'God, if there is anything I can say or not say to help this person in her journey—I am listening.'"

*—A caregiver*

"Wife: My buns show! I hate hospital gowns. How can I be decent and dignified wearing this horrid thing? I never thought I would be so dependent on someone else for the most intimate elements of my daily, personal care. You are my dear husband and I love being intimate with you—but not this way. You have been so wonderful through all of this. Thank you. I am so grateful that you and these wonderful nurses are here to do what I can't do for myself.

"Husband: You are so very welcome. It has been a hard journey together but I guess this is the part of the wedding vows about for better and for worse. Yes, this has been the longest and the worst we have ever endured. But, on the other hand, I'm thankful that I still enjoy looking at your beautiful buns."

*—A wife and caregiver husband.*

"Yes, I know a little something about never expecting your life to go a particular way, and still being able to make lemonade with it. It's a real choice, isn't it? And not always such an easy one, I have to say. After years of fighting this disease, and the frustrations and seeming unfairness of growing up in my family complete with the scars and post-traumatic stress disorder to prove it, only to then get diagnosed with a progressive disease as soon as I got free of there, I found myself saying aloud: 'I would have never known how loved I was if I had never had this disease. I never would have stopped overworking, and I would have continued to believe that whatever love and kindness came my way would have been because of what I was doing, and not who I was being.'

"Would I prefer to have it a different way? As teenagers say, 'Helllll yes!' But there has come to be some sort of peace about what is, and a kind of a gratitude for the days that are good ones—and hopefully, at least, some sense of humor about the other ones."

*—A grateful care receiver*

"The world is so full of care and sorrow that it is a gracious debt we owe to one another to discover the bright crystals of delight hidden in the somber circumstances and irksome tasks."

*—Helen Keller*

"No one is as capable of gratitude as one who has emerged from the kingdom of night."

*—Elie Wiesel in accepting the Nobel Peace Prize in 1986*

"O Lord, that lends me life,
Lend me a heart replete with thankfulness!"

*—William Shakespeare*

"There are two kinds of gratitude: the sudden kind we feel for what we receive, and the larger kind we feel for what we give."

*—Poet Edward Arlington Robinson*

## Let's Get Your Spirit Ready for a New Day

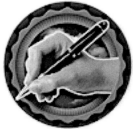

Name two positive effects resulting from being a caregiver of your beloved. Many have been surprised by this request. Their initial response has been that there is nothing positive about it. Upon further reflection, they have recorded some positive realities such as always having a purpose for living.

In groups, I get responses like: "I have defined my purpose and meaning for life" or "I always have a reason to get up in the morning. I may not want to get up but I do because I always have a reason to get up."

Write your answer, but make it short.

Try to go a step further. Now name two positive contributions of this situation on your spiritual and religious life.

## Let's Imagine

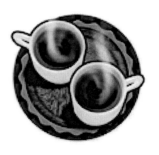

The weather has turned quite cold and blustery. A hint of winter is definitely in the air. It should be— Thanksgiving is soon upon us. We are huddled in the corner with our hot coffee. This time I have ordered my bagel with lox, cream cheese, capers and red onion. You keep teasing me about the way I order my bagels.

Then, I say, "I've been thinking about the prayers of those who will gather around our table for Thanksgiving. With unemployment still high, foreclosures, two war fronts, people in our country slipping below the poverty level without enough food for the Thanksgiving dinner, our planet groaning under the weight of our misuse of resources, there is so much to pray for. Then there are the families like ours with a caregiver and a care receiver.

"This year, I think we'll see three types of prayers. Some people, of course, will give thanks that things aren't worse than they are in their personal lives. Some will give thanks for the blessings they have received. Then, as Edward Arlington Robinson suggested, a few will give thanks for what they are able to give.

"Something significant has been happening within me lately, I'm moving more toward this last position. There is a shift that I feel deep within me: I have come to accept that my beloved will always live with her condition and it will affect both of us. I don't fight it anymore. I seem to have embraced that this is our shared fate. I have accepted the losses. I am free to be more responsive to her and others in a more gracious manner."
You respond...

# CHAPTER 21

# Laughing

## My Voice...

Caregivers know that their day-to-day tasks can represent the difference between life and death for a loved one. If you are reading this guidebook, then you know the serious nature of the challenges we face.

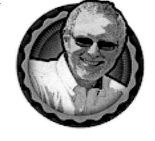

But now it's time to say: Don't take yourself too seriously! We may be the only ones available as caregivers for our loved ones at the moment, but we're not the only people on the planet who can perform these tasks. Let's be honest. I'm not God and neither are you—thank God! Did you know that humor is part of most of the world's great spiritual traditions? The Indian-born filmmaker Mira Nair made a half-hour documentary about "laughing clubs" in India that get together regularly for the healthy, yoga-like discipline of guffawing in unison.

Do you doubt there's any humor in your life? Have you ever started honestly swapping stories of your foibles with a friend? Ever tried sharing tales of flat-out flubs? How about our eccentricities? Soon, we're laughing and that is very healthy for us—and everyone around us.

Laughter tames fear, as so many bright people have pointed out down through the centuries. Laughter reduces stress. A belly-shaking explosion of laughter can blot out time and anxiety. You know how to get your computer going again when it slows to a crawl from an accumulation of too many programs whizzing through its brain. Well, think of laughter as rebooting the body and soul.

So, let's get serious about our need for humor!

# Wisdom of the Community...

"A good laugh and a long sleep are the best cures in the doctor's book."

  *—Irish Proverb*

"God is a comedian playing to an audience that's too afraid to laugh."

  *—Attributed to several sages, including H.L. Mencken and Voltaire*

"Things are so sad, so terrible—if you didn't laugh, you'd kill yourself."

  *— Woody Allen*

"Tragedy is when I cut my finger.
Comedy is when you fall into an open sewer and die."

  *—Mel Brooks*

"Everything is funny as long as it is happening to somebody else."

  *— Will Rogers*

"Comedy is tragedy plus time."

  *—Carol Burnett*

"A day without laughter is like a day without sunshine."

  *—Charlie Chaplin*

"A laugh can be a very powerful thing. Why, sometimes in life, it's the only weapon we have."

   —*Roger Rabbit*

**Forced Bulbs**

*It's not funny—yet,*
*We smiled a stiff smile as the day unfolded—*
*It's not funny*
*to be told you may be*
*facing death*
*in the near future—But*
*we even joked as we*
*went to buy bulbs to*
*force birth*
*into our home—and*
*keep death at bay!!*

   —*Poem of a caregiver*

"Shred the invitation—the party is cancelled—no pity party today. I need to kick my self-pity in the butt and be useful in whatever way I can."

   —*A caregiver*

"Lots of things make me laugh. I love the two people who are my caregivers…they both make me laugh a lot. One time I thought I was going to fall out of my wheelchair, they had me laughing so much. I love going on walks. I love looking at people and noticing the small things about them. I like to see people pulled over for traffic violations…I don't know why but it makes me laugh. I love sitting and staring at the clouds…I guess I'm like Charlie

Brown and his friends naming the clouds. I laugh when I have friends over and I can cook for them."

*—A man living in a caregiving relationship*

"Oh, did I happen to mention: 'Shit Happens!' I remember when I first heard that phrase and my explosive response was, 'No Shit!' Never in all my life did I imagine I would have to clean up my father's body after he soiled himself. And then later I had to give him an enema. No shit! No Fun! Body fluids are no fun, no shit."

*—A caregiver*

"So let me get back to your question. How have I coped with being a caregiver of my spouse? Well, often not too well. Usually, though, those are the times I take myself too seriously. If I can keep a sense of humor, which, of course, is not taking myself too seriously, then I can get this very serious job done—Ha, Ha, I'm not so scared—and that's important. Maybe the most important thing is not to get too scared.

"Let me show you one example of how I do it. Out here in my laundry room I have a coffee mug filled with old-thin-almost-used-up bars of soap. They are just the right size to give my hands—or my mouth when necessary—a quick washing. See what the cup says: 'Make Me Late For Breakfast.' Early in our marriage we used to tease and seduce each other with that line early in the mornings. Then one day we found this cup and howled—we had to buy it. Both of us used the cup with coffee to attempt to seduce the other. We loved our sexual life together.

"Every time I see that cup I get a bit wistful. I also smile and tease myself that the soap is there to wash out my mouth if I curse what is lost. It's one of many small ways I practice attitude adjustment—to keep smiling and hanging in there."

—*A caregiver*

---

"I know that I take myself and what has happened in our family much too seriously. It is serious, but it can swamp me if I don't adjust to the reality that it is going to be this way for a long time. I need to smile more—even laugh out loud more—not easy considering the circumstances. So, one thing I have done is set up a few surprises that will usually bring a smile or even a laugh. I definitely need that to happen if I am going to stay sane and balanced in this lopsided life as a caregiver.

"I occasionally find a short statement that makes me laugh. Sometimes I just write it on my bathroom mirror in lipstick. That makes for a good way to start a day or even helps me when I'm out of bed to answer nature's call in the middle of the night. At other times, I will write the statement on a small piece of paper and may even crumple it and then hide it in an odd place—like a knife drawer, in my wallet between the ones or under my pillow. Oh, I know it sounds silly but so what! If it makes me chuckle in the midst of all of this, then it is good foolishness.

"Here are a few samples of what makes me chuckle. A couple of these hit so close to the bone that I never know if they will make me laugh or cry—but I always hope I'll laugh when I discover words like these:

"On the other hand…you have different fingers.

I just got lost in thought. It wasn't familiar territory.

I feel like I'm diagonally parked in a parallel universe.

The early bird may get the worm, but the second mouse gets the cheese.

Depression is merely anger without enthusiasm.

Remember—if the world did not suck, we would all fall off.

The shinbone is an appendage for finding furniture in a dark room.

Wrinkles are something others have, similar to my character lines.

When everything is coming your way, you're in the wrong lane.

Plan to be spontaneous tomorrow."

*—A caregiver*

---

"I cannot agree more about humor being a life and relationship saver. When people had to drive me everywhere because I could not put weight on either leg— **wow!** That was a bitch! I would send out the funniest, wickedest comments people had made about my 'unfetteredly' pitiful state with my weekly ride request emails called, 'The Ankle of the Week Awards.'

"Humor is as vital as oxygen. While I had to be in casts, I found the most ungodly garish, hilarious socks possible to wear visibly with the casts. It turns out they actually make socks big enough to fit fully grown women that have pink, purple and lime green pom-poms hanging off them. That right there? Waaayyy better than therapy.

"That, and friends bringing Play-Doh to the hospital and making 'voodoo' nurses to stick needles in on my hospital bedside table when I lost my kidney? Best medical intervention in my whole life! Then there was the giant rubber snake wrapped around my IV pole with the bloody fangs at the needle site.

"You cannot say enough about humor. And I think that humor gives people accessibility. The more people see themselves in my pom-pom socks, the less threatening my condition. That's true whether you're a caregiver or receiver. The fact that I could laugh at my ankle/wheel-chair predicament, and that others could too, made it much easier to ask for help with that than with my kidney disease.

"The more ooey-gooey the need/illness—breast cancer, prostate cancer, mental illness (so private, humbling and intimate)—the more freaked out we get. On both sides of the care relationship, I think. Humor can't level that playing field completely, but I think it at least provides an invitation into the conversation."

*—A woman in caregiving relationships*

---

"They laughed at each other's speech, with the brook that ran near them, and the laughter of Jesus was the merrier. And they conversed long."

*—Khalil Gibran*

---

"Without the laughter, there would be no Way."

*—Laozi/Lao-tzu in the Tao Te Ching*

---

"You can't laugh and be afraid at the same time."

*—Attributed to many writers, most recently Stephen Colbert*

---

"Laughter is the shortest distance between two people."

*—Victor Borge*

---

"Mirth is God's medicine. Everybody ought to bathe in it."

*—Henry Ward Beecher*

# Let's Get Your Spirit Ready for a New Day

Can you remember the last time you laughed? What was so funny? Have you told a friend?

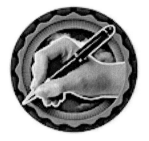

Jot down a few notes about a tender and tough moment in your life as a caregiver. Did it include a moment of humor?

Start your own strategy for humorous surprises. Where will you hide your funniest lines?

Ask your friends to make you a laugh envelope tailored just for you. They know what will make you laugh. When you need a little chuckle, pick one of the pages from the envelope and see if it makes you smile and lifts your spirit. Have a good laugh and then you might even want to call your friend—both of you will enjoy the moment. List the friends you will ask to help create your laugh envelope.

Host a laugh-in party. Admission: 1 joke. If anyone makes a negative comment: charge him or her one dollar! Give the money to your favorite advocacy group. Have a five-minute "whine-and-gripe" session in the middle of the laugh-in party and see how much laughter it creates.

Do any of the lines or ideas in this chapter tickle your funny bone? Add a few of your own funny lines or good ideas for laughter to our website . [www.GuideForCaregivers.info] .

Where will you hide some items or lines that will surprise and make you laugh? Try it: let yourself be foolish! Enjoy the chuckles.

# Let's Imagine

It is good to be back together again. We both seem eager to talk and even tease each other a bit. We really have become close in so many ways over these few months. For that, I think we are both quite grateful.

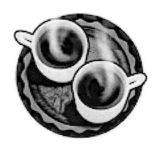

I say: "I'm 6' 4", with a scruffy beard, a wry smile, some vital muscles, still plenty of testosterone—and I always carry a tissue. Oh, yes, I use it for my own nose. After all, a tissue is for cold storage. Mainly, though, I carry them in my caregiver toolbox. A white flag of peace, a dauber for bodily fluids, a reminder that on this quiet battlefield, I need to keep my heart and soul peaceful with a touch—a sweeping touch—of wry, ironic humor and very pragmatic tools, like a tissue. Somebody! A tisssshhue, puh-leeease!!"

And I'm chuckling already.

You respond...

# CHAPTER 22

# Blessing

## My Voice...

There is a yearning in most of us for a word, a look, a touch that blesses us. A deep hunger within cries out for more than validation of our common humanity; we hunger for a word of grace. We want and need a declaration that we are known to our core, yet truly loved—not only for what we do—but who we are.

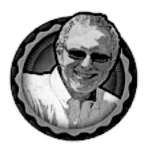

We hunger for someone who can look us in the eyes, knowing all our shortcomings, and still extend the bounty of their heart to embrace us with grace and gladness. We yearn for that blessing from another person and for that blessing from the One who gave us life and who will call us unto death.

A blessing is more than a religious benediction. A blessing is a gift that is shared and received with transforming tenderness and compassionate love. A blessing can be extended in a few caring words, a tender and warm touch, a look that embraces the soul.

Caregivers constantly have the power to extend a blessing, and we do.

But remember this above all: Caregivers need blessing, too. And, when those moments do surprise us—most of us have the humility to receive the gift we are given. May it be so with you.

# Wisdom of the Community...

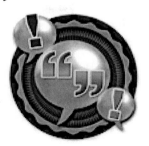

"Blessed are the poor in spirit; for theirs is the kingdom of heaven."

> —*Jesus*

"A person of truth—must also be a person of care."

> —*Gandhi*

## Holding Environment (For Judith and Ben)

*"I would like to come and hold you:*
*You, who have yourselves held so many*
*As they struggled with life—*
*And death.*

*I would like to come and hold you,*
*And let you be, in my arms,*
*Sad, silent, angry, confused*
*As your heart dictates*
*Moment to moment.*

*I would like to come and hold you,*
*Wagering on God's grace*
*Until S/He wipes away every tear*
*From your eyes—*
*And from mine;*
*And builds a new Jerusalem,*
*A kin-dom,*
*In our hearts.*

*I would like to come and hold you,*
*But I hesitate. . .*
*For to be thus held is to become*

A little child all over again,
And that's a hoped-for-but-resisted
Birth
Which always feels like dying.
Forceps are contraindicated, for it's
A leaving terrifying in its inevitability,
Painful in its process,
Threatening to that prowess
By which each day is lived.
And there's been enough of that
Already.

I would like to come and hold you,
And will if it's your wish.
But I will also stand at a distance
Quietly
Remembering my losses and my
Births-that-feel-like-death
So that I might mingle my experiences
With yours in
Laughter and sadness at this
Mystery
We keep flipping into the air,
Praying it will always come up
Heads.
(Las Vegas reports a 50-50 chance of
Tails.)

I would like to come and hold you,
And together be embraced
By the One for whom
Heads and tails define
The only coins S/He made;
And in whose arms, in time,
All our losses

*Are changed to winnings,*
*All our tears to joy."*

    *—James M. Truxell, February 23, 1993*

---

"I wish you not a path devoid of clouds,
Nor a life on a bed of roses,
Nor that you might never need regret,
Nor that you should never feel pain.
My wish for you is:
That you might be brave in times of trial...
When hope scarce can shine through.
That every gift God gave you might grow along with you
And let you give the gift of joy to all who care for you.
That you may always have a friend who is worth that name,
Whom you can trust, and who helps you in times of sadness,
Who will defy the storms of daily life at your side.
One more wish I have for you:
That in every hour of joy and pain
You may feel God close to you.
This is my wish for you, now and forever.
Amen."

    *—A Celtic blessing*

---

"I know I'm doing mostly OK when something simple makes
me smile inside as well as with my eyes and lips:
A pleasant song is repeating in my head as I awaken for the
day
A woodpecker pecks away at the suet feeder and my heart
flutters with delight
A sudden burst of sunlight casts a golden glow off our yellow
wall and I feel bathed in warmth
A quick call from our daughter makes me feel loved
A dear friend shows up at the door with matzo ball soup

*Simple blessings remind me of love, hope, gratitude and the basic blessings and goodness of life as it is given. I return to my extraordinarily ordinary and ordinarily extraordinary tasks of caregiving with a lighter and more purposeful heart."*

*—A caregiver*

## Holding Hands at 3 A.M.

*"I awaken at 3 a.m.*
*We are holding hands*
*I squeeze gently—don't want to awaken her*
*—she squeezes a gentle response.*
*No words spoken—nothing to say—*
*it is all being said with*
*our hands at*
*3 a.m.*
*Yes—we are here for*
*each other!"*

*—A caregiver awaiting a cancer diagnosis*

"It is love that asks, that seeks, that knocks, that finds, and that is faithful to what it finds."

*—Augustine of Hippo*

"It takes courage to love, but pain through love is the purifying fire which those who love generously know."

*—Eleanor Roosevelt*

"When you stop giving and offering something to the rest of the world—it's time to turn out the lights."

*—George Burns*

### A Blessing for Caregivers

*"Create in all caregivers a clean heart, O God, and put a new, courageous and resilient spirit within each through community, presence, grieving, gratitude, music, humor and disciplines of heart, mind and body.*

*Teach caregivers that you weep when you see their sacrifice. Protect caregivers from a bitter and cynical heart. Surely, You will not reject a humble and repentant heart, O God.*

*Embrace and instill within caregivers love, generosity, courage, good will and grace.*

*O Creator God, be tender in shaping us.*

*O Loving God, bless us in your own eternal compassion. Amen."*

—*Adapted from a portion of Psalm 51*

---

# Let's Get Your Spirit Ready for a New Day

Do you hunger for a blessing?

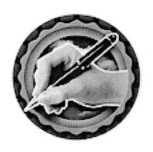

Do you know that you have the power to give a blessing?

Who will bless you today? How will the blessing come?

Who will you bless today? Will you do it with a word, a cup of water or tea, a note, a touch or a tender look?

Describe the last time you gave or received Grace.

# PART 6

## Resources

# CHAPTER 23

# Forming a Group

## Forming a Small Storytelling Group

Why is it so important to tell our stories to others? Many scholars have offered answers, but here's the best answer: It changes lives. We tell our stories to strangers on airplanes, to therapists, in AA groups and, occasionally, in our marriages and families. Sometimes, we do it because we read a book like this one.

This book can be used for individual or group study. If you keep this process solely to yourself, you can fall into one of the traps we urge you to avoid: Don't do the job alone. If you work through these ideas in a group, be careful: You still want to process all of this individually as well. You may choose to write down your story, but remember—that's not the same as telling your story to listeners who respond with eyes and hearts as you talk and who can form relationships with you in an ongoing way.

In this portion of the "Resources" section, I'm offering just one of many possible ways to structure a small group. You can use this entire book as a guide for discussion as you see fit. But consider the following ideas for a storytelling group. Such a group could help you clarify your own story, learn why you are struggling in some areas and not in others as a caregiver, and liberate you for a new perspective and understanding of yourself.

First, let me share a few thoughts about the formation of a group.

A group does not make a community. Community is formed when we have shared and listened to each other's stories and have become aware that there is a common story that unites us.

The primary purpose of this group is to learn from telling and listening to common stories. The members are the resources. Storytelling is the curriculum. Storytelling is the surest way of touching human spirits and forming the bonds necessary to create community.

One important truth I have learned in such groups is: Space out your meetings. For example, if you design a six-week series, consider taking two weeks off between each two-week segment of meetings. The value in this is that it gives each person time and space to process the intensity of their own and others' stories. I cannot overemphasize how important this is to the process.

The optimal size of a group is 8-12 people. But please remember that community can be formed where two or three are gathered in trust-filled sharing.

Decisions need to be made among the participants about confidentiality, leadership, place and time, and schedule of meetings. I urge you to set the standard at "what-is-said-in-this-room-stays-in-this-room— **period** !" The millions of Americans familiar with 12-step programs understand why that kind of rule is so helpful.

## Choosing a Group Leader

Here are a few suggestions when choosing a group leader.

If you choose to invite or designate a leader, the leader needs to understand that she is not present as a group member seeking to solve and deal with her own issues. The leader should be a seasoned caregiver, not in crisis, and be clear that her presence is as the leader. You may want a faith leader, a pastoral counselor, a social worker or someone skilled in group leadership. You may need to pay a leader.

Choose a leader who can and will set good boundaries. The leader must emphasize an economy of words and time as the group members tell their stories. People who are under stress, anxiety and turmoil are prone to talking excessively and repetitively or to withdrawing into silence. A leader will be empathically present, but capable of maintaining emotional and physical distance.

A good leader will enable storytellers to deepen their story with new and fresh insight and meaning.

Choose a leader for the group who is more interested in listening and hearing than in talking. A good leader will facilitate the process of storytelling and will aide in the interpretation of stories.

# Becoming a Good Listener

"If one gives answer before he hears, it is his folly and shame."
—*Proverbs 18:13*

The truth be told, most of us are hungry to be heard. We often make our conversations into competitive matches that no one wins. Our competitive urge is paralleled by a fear response: "I don't know what to say when he talks about such difficult things." Since we don't understand that attentive silence is a powerful form of speech, we yammer away into another subject as a competitive distraction.

Good listeners are hard to find. The number one attribute and gift of a good listener is not the ear; it is the heart—a loving, hospitable heart. Hospitality means having enough love to welcome a friend or stranger, and to be more interested in that person than in one's self and one's own agenda. Hospitality makes space to truly listen to the other's story.

Hospitality requires only discerning comments as one listens. It invites clarification. It does not offer judgment or advice. A hospitable listener wants to know the whole story and assist by quietly inviting details. This is where the artistry of listening comes into play. Especially valuable is the ability to hear the story beneath the spoken words, to sense the message in the speaker's eyes as they silently convey volumes, then to invite the teller to voice the unspoken.

# Preparing to Tell Your Story: the Short, Core Story

Our identity rests in our story. For most of us, our primary story was crafted in early life and often forms a script for the way we live our lives now. Our story shapes our choice of relationships with life partners, our vocations and our approaches to parenting.

To prepare for a storytelling group, it's valuable to start by jotting down a very short version of your core story. Here is how I capture my own story in one sentence:

My mother became an invalid because I was born.

That one sentence tells you very little about the course of my entire life—but it tells you a lot about the powerful influences shaping my life. I can spell out my life's story in much greater depth, but—when all is said and done—my gifts and blessings, my curses and limitations all stem from that core story.

Here are examples of other core stories I've heard in groups:

- "I was born on third base. Of course I want you to think I hit a triple. "

- "Both my parents were alcoholics. I never knew what normal was! "

- "Responsibility. It was the word and the action of my parents. I was always to be responsible in everything I said and did. "

- "I think I was an accident that no one wanted. I always dreamed that some prince would rescue me and love me just for me. "

- "My ministerial father only wanted sons. He wanted a boy who could become a minister in his conservative, "no ordained women allowed" church. So, when I was born a girl, my role was to marry a minister. I did. "

- "I have always been competitive. I had to be the best. Perfect was the only choice. "

- "I have always been a whiner. I seemed to be sad and angry at the same time, so I combined them: I whined. I was never satisfied. "

Got the idea? Write your own short, core story. But, please, be gentle with yourself. It may take longer than you think to write this clearly and honestly. Let it unfold—quietly and tenderly.

Can't do it in one sentence? Well, take five or six—but no more than a paragraph.

## Preparing to Tell Your Story: the Longer Story

Life comes at us with many offerings of opportunities, contingencies, joys and sorrows. The way we respond to what life gives us is viewed and shaped through our core story. The way we handle our relationships, our work, our marriages, our children, our parents is, in some way, impacted by that story.

If you are reading this book, your life has been deeply affected by becoming a caregiver for someone who lives with physical, emotional, mental or intellectual limitations. This is now a major part of the story you are living.

After writing your core story—try writing your longer story.

You may wonder why it is important for you to write this story when it is so much a part of your bones. You could attend your storytelling group and simply let your story flow. However, spending time in writing your own story can clarify lots of things as you commit your experiences to words. You'll be surprised by the connections you may make and how the choices of words can shape your understanding of what you've experienced.

One major reason to write your story is that you're planning to tell it in your group. As you write, envision members of your group and imagine yourself talking to them. Writing down this longer version of your story will help you tell a concise version of your story without falling into so many digressions that your group leader will call "time" before you've finished what you're eager to say.

Just how long should this "longer story" be when you are finished? Try to keep it to a single page if you are typing it out on your computer.

Or, here's another way to describe that goal: Keep it to several paragraphs if you're writing with a pen on a pad or in a blank-page book. With three paragraphs, you can devote the first one to basic background about your family; the second can describe your personal responsibilities in this situation; and the third can describe your thoughts and feelings about it all.

Again, be tender with yourself and let this unfold gently.

# CHAPTER 24

# Understanding Burnout and Accidie

## Burnout

More than a century ago, Emily Dickinson wrote:

*I measure every grief I meet*
*With analytic eyes;*
*I wonder if it weighs like mine,*
*Or has an easier size.*

*I wonder if they bore it long,*
*Or did it just begin?*
*I could not tell the date of mine*
*It feels so old a pain.*

*I wonder if it hurts to live,*
*And if they have to try,*
*And whether could they choose between,*
*They would not rather die.*

The cry I hear from countless caregivers, even professionals, is far less eloquent than Dickinson's lines. Usually, they cry one word: "Burnout!" They have either experienced it or are heading in that direction. Doctors, nurses, clergy, educators, police, fire and rescue personnel—all whose profession involves caregiving—are at risk. Burnout is the central issue for family and friends who have dedicated their lives to their loved one who will never be fully independent. Where does our initial fire go? What drenches the flames of our passion to help?

What is burnout? Let's look at what it is not. Burnout is not just exhaustion and fatigue. What it is is weariness, frustration and loss of energy brought about by the failure of idealized assumptions. As our dreams fade, we lose our passion and energy, and the fire goes out. We are burned out!

Death Valley was once an ocean teaming with life. Refreshing water flowed into and out of this sea, vitalizing the sea and the area around it. Then geologic shifts challenged and changed the landscape and threatened the life of the ocean. The waters that fed the sea stopped flowing, but the outflow continued. The sea gave away all that it had. It dried up and became a desert. The once life-giving sea no longer existed. Without refreshing water it died, resulting in Death Valley.

This can be an alarmingly accurate metaphor of caregivers' lives. The time when you become fully aware that your loved one is under your care is like a geologic shift in the landscape of your world. All of your vitality flows outward and very little flows in to refresh you. You yearn for a trickle of refreshing water to restore your sense of vitality—physically, emotionally, relationally, and spiritually. You give, sacrifice and empty yourself with little or no time or energy directed toward receiving—or even taking—what you need for yourself.

There are two umbrella issues invariably present in burnout—distribution and expectation. The distribution issue is illustrated by the Death Valley metaphor. Expectation describes the goal-oriented idealism of many caregivers. We have a vision for our marriage, our family, our congregation, our country, our employer and our children. In every area of our lives, reality can be shocking. We are prone to measuring our lives by the accomplishment of our expectations. When they are not fulfilled, we feel disoriented and dislodged, baffled and defeated.

Others may see many of the warning signs of burnout before they are recognized by the victim. The most insidious and devastating aspect of burnout is the way that it gradually consumes a person over an extended period of time.

Is burnout the same as stress? Stress is the non-specific psychological and physiological response to events that are believed and perceived to be a threat to one's well being. Burnout is the drying-up of our resources due to excessive striving based on unrealistic expectations and a failure to replenish these resources. The key element is that stress relates to beliefs and perceptions; burnout relates to expectations.

Burnout is the result of a failure to balance the distribution of our energy by refueling ourselves with the healing waters that will enable us to continue our difficult work as caregivers. This book is primarily a guide to restoring ourselves after burnout or avoiding it altogether.

I invite you to do a difficult but necessary exercise. Briefly describe one of your dreams that has been deferred or has dried up as a consequence of your caregiving relationship. Of course, you are free to list more than one if it benefits you. Be very specific.

Consider these questions:

- Has the disruption of your dream made you sad, mad, had, glad or numb?
- What positive came from the disruption of your dream?

Yes, you read that second question correctly. We usually learn more from *not* getting what we want. Our stumbling blocks can become life's building blocks. Burnout does not always produce a negative outcome. It may be the occasion for us to become more fully aware of ourselves, wrestle with our value system, grieve our failed dreams and readjust our priorities. Then, we can revise and reenvision our dreams. Burnout can be a time to start a reorienting dialogue with God and others. Yes, we can experience burnout as a dismembering of our ego, but this may be necessary to get our attention and remake us as more functional and loving beings. Yes, it will feel as if we are losing the self and life we have known. But, this is a time when we must give up our omnipotent and idealized visions—we are free to begin a new pilgrimage of holiness and wholeness. If you take this paragraph seriously, you'll want to pay particular attention to sections on grieving and thanking in this book.

Are you burned out? Here's a little mental exercise to try at home. Go stand just outside your kitchen in an adjoining room. Close your eyes and picture in your mind's eye that you are lifting one leg slowly to let it reach forward until you enter the kitchen. Don't actually do it—this exercise is about using your imagination to envision a simple action. You may want to laugh, and that is appropriate since this seems like a silly exercise. But it's also very serious, because burnout can destroy your imagination and playfulness which are so necessary to envision slowly stepping into another room—or to begin revitalizing your life.

Next, try a more comforting and serious exercise of the imagination—not necessarily at this moment, but soon. When you have 10 to 15 minutes of privacy, go into a quiet area and sit in a very comfortable chair. Picture the person who brings you the greatest comfort and solace in your life. Picture yourself sitting in his or her lap in a rocking chair. No words, no gestures, just a time when you, the caregiver, will be rocked and comforted. Let yourself soak in the comfort and solace.

# Accidie

Accidie is the spiritual word most closely aligned with burnout. Accidie (´ak-sə-dē)—also sometimes written as acedia (ə-´sē-dē- ə)—comes from the Greek word *akedos* that refers to those who didn't care enough to bury the dead on the battlefield—those who had the passion for battle but became indifferent because of such great loss. Accidie was translated in the Middle Ages by its symptoms: sloth or torpor. But these symptoms inadequately describe the root meaning of this potent word that refers to spiritual dryness or spiritual suicide. In its fullest meaning, accidie refers to the loss of joy or faith in the goodness of life or the goodness of God.

Accidie is the evil of indifference and boredom lightly coated with cynicism. It leaves one passionless, apathetic and with no taste for life. Our spirits are broken. We function without any great delight and joy in our lives.

It is easy to get mired in the difficult parts of our life story. Our dreams are not working out, yet we hold on to them. It is too frightening to let go of them because they are the foundation of our lives. We hang onto our anger because it is better than letting go and falling into the abyss of the unknown. Without letting go of dead dreams, we cannot mourn their loss. The anger to which we cling congeals into resentment. Beneath the anger and resentment is sadness beyond sorrow that brings us to the brink of a broken spirit—accidie.

When Dante descends to the Fifth Circle of the Inferno in *The Divine Comedy* , he finds a black and loathsome marsh made by the dark waters of the Stygian stream which pours into it. There, in the putrid swamp, he sees the souls of those whom anger has ruined. They are hitting, tearing and maiming one another in ceaseless, senseless rage. But there are others there, the Master tells him, whom he cannot see—whose sobs make bubbles that rise to the surface. Who are these others and how are they ruined by anger? Fixed in the slime, they say: "Sullen were we in the sweet air, that is gladdened by the sun, carrying lazy smoke within our hearts, now lie we sullen here in the black mire," Dante tells us. This hymn they gurgle in their throats, for they cannot speak in full words. It is a hymn of burnout.

Dante is describing people drowning in accidie, too. His powerful words provide us with an early and clear portrayal of how we become mired in the muck of life, as well as what happens to us once we get stuck there. Claiming unbroken sullenness and willful gloom as key elements to getting "fixed in the slime," Dante declares that people in this condition can't even speak but are left to "gurgle."

The loss of dreams usually comes in two ways: mirror-shattering events or foundation-eroding experiences. Whether quick or slow, these losses wound our core identity. We have worked hard, dreamed hard, played hard, fought hard, yet our story has not turned out like the script. We have believed in our government, fought for our country, and worshipped in our synagogues, mosques, and churches only to find that these institutions have clay feet. We have devoted ourselves to family, marriage, children, and the pursuit of the good life only to discover that the living reality is considerably more limited than our idyllic dreams. We find ourselves disappointed, despairing of the outcome, and bone-weary. That is the pathway to accidie.

The weariness of which I speak is not the normal weariness of a hard day in the field, factory, office or home. It is a weariness of the heart and the spirit that comes from being tired of what is and being without hope for what is to come. We see this weariness on our faces from time to time when we stare into the mirror. We recognize the look in the subway, the office and even at the ballpark. It is the look that reveals how difficult living can be and how we wish we could find a haven where we wouldn't ache anymore—where the weariness would be taken away and where we could stop holding our breath and exhale.

Two authors published books on accidie only months apart in 2008. I published *Ian Fleming's Seven Deadlier Sins & 007's Moral Compass* . Chapter 007 focuses on accidie in our lives. *Acedia & me* , by Kathleen Norris, is an encyclopedic exploration of this subject.

# CHAPTER 25

# Reading to Revive the Soul

## Online

Please visit our website [www.GuideForCaregivers.info] for much more about caregiving, recommendations of groups that are working across the country to help individuals and families with these challenges—and helpful articles by myself and other writers. Over time, that website will expand to help a wide range of people, especially if you will take the time to visit it and add some of your own ideas as suggested throughout this book.

## Other Recommended Books

- Mitch Albom. *Tuesdays with Morrie: An Old Man, a Young Man and Life's Greatest Lesson.*
- Rosalynn Carter. *Helping Yourself Help Others, A Book for Caregivers.*
- Joan Chittister. *Wisdom Distilled from the Daily, Living the Rule of St. Benedict Today.*
- Wendell Berry. *Hannah Coulter: A Novel .*
- Tara Birch. *Radical Acceptance, Embracing Your Life with the Heart of a Buddha.*
- Ian Brown. *The Boy in the Moon, A Father's Journey to Understand His Extraordinary Son.*
- Frederick Buechner. *Now and Then, A Memoir of Vocation.*
- ---. *Listening to Your Life, Daily Meditations with Frederick Buechner.*

- ---. *The Sacred Journey, A Memoir of Early Days* .
- Jack Canfield. *Chicken Soup for the Soul* .
- Richard Carlson and Benjamin Shield. *Handbook for the Soul* .
- Kate DiCamilo. *The Miraculous Journey of Edward Tulane* .
- Wayne Dyer. *Your Sacred Self, Making the Decision to Be Free* .
- Margaret Edson. *Wit, A Play* .
- Matthew Fox. *Original Blessing, A Primer in Creation Spirituality Presented in Four Paths, Twenty-Six Themes and Two Questions.*
- Robert Fulghum. *All I Really Need to Know I Learned in Kindergarten* .
- Graham Greene. *The Burnt-Out Case* .
- Olga Grushin. *The Line* .
- The Brothers Halamandaris. *Caring Quotes, A Compendium of Caring Thought* .
- Gerald G. Jampolsky, M.D. *Love Is Letting Go of Fear* .
- Ernest Kurtz and Katherine Ketcham. *The Spirituality of Imperfection, Storytelling and the Search for Meaning.*
- Yann Martel. *Life of Pi* .
- Ian McEwan. *Saturday* .
- Donald Miller . *Searching for God Knows What* .
- Henry Nouwen . *Adam, God's Beloved* .
- ---. *Our Greatest Gift, A Meditation on Dying and Caring* .
- ---. *The Inner Voice of Love, A Journey Through Anguish to Freedom* .
- ---. *The Return of the Prodigal Son, A Story of Homecoming* .
- Wayne E. Oates. *Nurturing Silence in a Noisy Heart* .

- Jodi Picoult. *My Sister's Keeper, A Novel* .
- Susan Rava. *Swimming Solo* .
- Gail Sheehy. *Passages in Caregiving, Turning Chaos into Confidence.*
- Michael A. Singer. *The Untethered Soul, The Journey Beyond Yourself* .
- Lewis B. Smedes. *The Art of Forgiving, When You Need to Forgive and Don't Know How.*
- Barbara Brown Taylor. *An Altar in the World, A Geography of Faith* .
- Marjorie J. Thompson. *Soul Feast, An Invitation to the Christian Spiritual Life* .
- Anne Tyler. *Saint Maybe* .
- Catherine Whitmire. *Plain Living, A Quaker Path to Simplicity* .
- William P. Young. *The Shack, Where Tragedy Confronts Eternity* .

# Acknowledgements

DURING THE WRITING OF this book, I have received encouragement, support and teaching from numerous organizations—nonprofit as well as government—and from caregivers themselves and individuals who provide support for caregivers. I have attended classes for professional and informal caregivers. I have conducted numerous interviews and listened to conversations among caregivers.

I felt encouragement wherever I went during this long journey. Occasionally, I would mention in public that I was crafting a book about the care of caregivers and even strangers who overheard me would say: "Oh, I have good friends who are serving that way—with their child, parent, spouse, neighbor or friend."

I have chosen not to list names of the numerous contributors in order to protect their privacy. To each person and organization, I wish to extend sincere and heartfelt thanks. You gave a gift to me personally and to the readers of this book with your honesty and candor.

I do want to acknowledge my soul brother, Jim Truxell. He, too, has been a caregiver, a pastoral counselor and a poet. We have loved, labored and laughed together for almost fifty years—teaching, cajoling and appreciating each other nearly every step of the way. Jim has given me permission to include three of his poems in this work. Thank you, my brother.

# About the Author

DR. BENJAMIN PRATT, A retired United Methodist Pastoral Counselor, has spent much of the last seven years in a care-giving relationship with Judith, his wife of 48 years. The book reflects his gleanings from his successes, trials and failures as a caregiver, a pastor and a professional counselor. They reside in Fairfax, Virginia.

# Colophon

READ THE SPIRIT BOOKS produces its titles using innovative digital systems that serve the emerging wave of readers who want their books delivered in a wide range of formats—from traditional print to digital readers in many shapes and sizes. This book was produced using this entirely digital process that separates the core content of the book from details of final presentation, a process that increases the flexibility and accessibility of the book's text and images. At the same time, our system ensures a well-designed, easy-to-read experience on all reading platforms, built into the digital data file itself.

David Crumm Media has built a unique production workflow employing a number of XML (Extensible Markup Language) technologies. This workflow, allows us to create a single digital "book" data file that can be delivered quickly in all formats from traditionally bound print-on-paper to digital screens.

During production, we use Adobe InDesign®, <Oxygen/>® XML Editor and Microsoft Word® along with custom tools built in-house.

The print edition is set in Minion Pro and Myriad Pro typefaces.

Cover art and Design by Rick Nease: www.RickNeaseArt.com.

Editing by David Crumm.

Copy editing and XML styling by Celeste Dykas.

Digital encoding and print layout by John Hile.

If you enjoyed this book, you may also enjoy

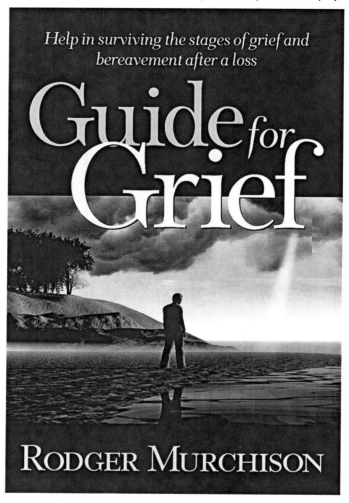

In his new Guide for Grief, the Rev. Rodger Murchison brings years of pastoral experience and study, sharing recommendations from both scripture and the latest research into loss and bereavement.

*http://www.GuideForGrief.com*

*ISBN: 978-1-934879-31-3*

If you enjoyed this book, you may also enjoy

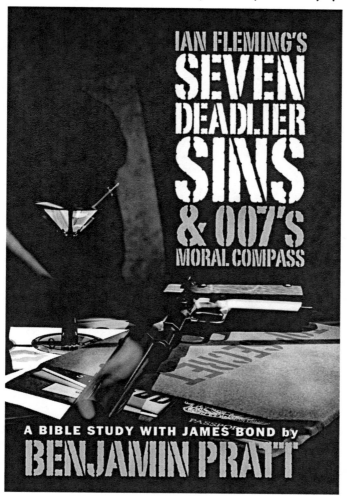

Here's a book that will reward your efforts as you look at evil through the eyes of Ian Fleming's James Bond. Like Bond, you too might be roused to take on the dragons of evil in our midst.

*http://www.JamesBondBibleStudy.com*

*ISBN: 978-1-934879-11-5*

If you enjoyed this book, you may also enjoy

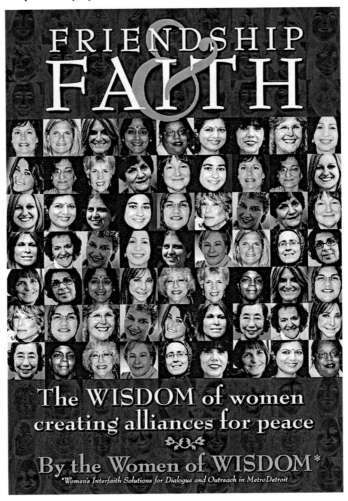

Finding a good friend is hard. Preserving a friendship across religious and cultural boundaries—a challenge we all face in our rapidly changing world—is even harder.

*http://www.FriendshipAndFaith.com*

*ISBN: 978-1-934879-19-1*

If you enjoyed this book, you may also enjoy

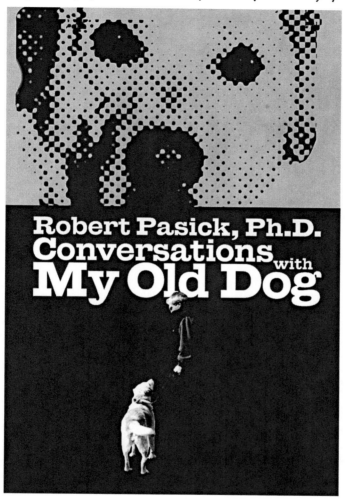

"Subtle doses of humor will bring a smile to your face. Maybe pets really do have solutions to life's perplexities!"

*—An Amazon Reviewer*

*http://www.ConversationsWithMyOldDog.com*

*ISBN: 978-1-934879-17-7*

CPSIA information can be obtained at www.ICGtesting.com
Printed in the USA
BVOW040155061011

272931BV00001B/5/P